John Little spent 25 years working as a reporter and producer in television current affairs before becoming a full-time author. He has written eight books, including *The Hospital by the River* (with Dr Catherine Hamlin); *Down to the Sea*; *Jem, a Father's Story*; *Christine's Ark*; and *Maalika* (with Valerie Browning). He lives with his wife, Anna, and son, Tim, on Sydney's northern beaches.

jdlittle@bigpond.com
www.johnlittle.info

CATHERINE'S GIFT

STORIES OF HOPE FROM THE HOSPITAL BY THE RIVER

JOHN LITTLE

MONARCH
BOOKS
Oxford, UK & Grand Rapids, Michigan, USA

First published in the UK in 2010 by Monarch Books
(a publishing imprint of Lion Hudson plc),
Wilkinson House, Jordan Hill Road, Oxford OX2 8DR.
Tel: +44 (0)1865 302750 Fax: +44 (0)1865 302757
Email: monarch@lionhudson.com
www.lionhudson.com

ISBN: 978-1-85424-955-5

Distributed by:
UK: Marston Book Services Ltd, PO Box 269, Abingdon, Oxon
OX14 4YN;
USA: Kregel Publications, PO Box 2607, Grand Rapids, Michigan
49501

British Library Cataloguing Data
A catalogue record for this book is available from the British Library.

Printed and bound in England by J. F. Print Ltd.

Once again, this one's for Anna

Every gift of noble origin
Is breathed upon by Hope's perpetual breath.

WILLIAM WORDSWORTH

PROLOGUE

It's the rainy season in Addis Ababa. The day begins with a promise. At the hospital by the river, patients who are not confined to bed throw off their woollen shawls and gather in the sun to gossip. The girls groom one another's hair, sew and bicker and joke. Some, perhaps speaking a rare tongue, sit by themselves on the low stone wall by the outpatients department, or squat on the ground watching the activity. In this self-contained little world, walled off from the chaos of the city, there's always something to see – new patients arriving, mud-stained, stinking and weary after travelling on foot over flooded tracks, vehicles bringing medical supplies, *ferenji* visitors from another planet, gardeners tending the lawns and flower beds, workers regularly hosing away the puddles which gather under the waiting patients.

These are peasant women. The seasons rule their lives. They savour the morning warmth, for they know that by midday black clouds will begin to form over the hills which ring the city and the thunder will grumble like a cranky old man leaving a warm bed. At two-thirty the rain begins – they could set their watches by it if they owned such things – and it does not stop until late at night.

1

In the highlands where many of these women come from, the rains can cut off villages for weeks on end. When doctors Reg and Catherine Hamlin first began treating the women half a century ago they could always count on some respite at this time of year. But for the past few years the rainy season seems to have made no difference. Is it because there are more cases than ever? Or just because the hospital has become so well known? Whatever the reason, every day up to half a dozen women arrive seeking help.

Sometimes they are alone – bewildered and frightened by the brutal indifference of the city. Sometimes a friend or relative has come with them. A few, with injuries so severe they are unable to walk, are carried in. They come from the desert, from remote highland villages, from the plains and the rainforest. They speak 80 different languages. They are Orthodox Christians, Muslims, Animists, or sometimes a mixture of faiths. They all have one thing in common – they are suffering from the medical condition known as obstetric fistula.

It is a cruel affliction. Ethiopia has its lepers and cripples, as does any poor African country. The diseased and the lame and the mad are on any street corner for all to see. But if there is a scale of human misery, the fistula women are up near the top. Imagine, if you will, how life would be as a woman whose bodily wastes leak out constantly through the vagina – a vile-smelling trickle which you were unable to control.

They believe they are cursed by God. And you have to wonder what God had in mind when he allowed a woman's most cherished act, childbirth, to produce this outcome. No matter where they live, 10 per cent of all women will experience some kind of problem, such as obstructed labour, during childbirth. In the west they simply go to hospital and have a caesarean section or a forceps delivery. For a peasant girl in a remote Ethiopian village it's not so easy. She will squat in her circular hut, or tukul, sometimes for days, trying to force the baby out. After a couple of days the baby inevitably dies. The prolonged labour, with the baby stuck in the birth canal, may cut off the blood supply to parts of the mother's body. The tissue dies, leaving a hole, or fistula, in the bladder, and sometimes the rectum.

Because they are so offensive to be near, fistula sufferers are invariably divorced by their husbands and banished from their village. Theirs are lives of loneliness and despair, often in some ruined dwelling away from everyone else, or they may be forced to beg for a living in the town. We are not talking about some minor medical curiosity here. There are 200,000 fistula sufferers in Ethiopia; two million throughout the world.

Amid the comings and goings, some of the girls may notice a tall, slim, grey-haired woman wearing a white doctor's coat, passing through the outpatients department into the main ward. Dr Catherine Hamlin is 83 now. She was 35 when she and her husband, Reg, also an obstetrician/gynaecologist, first came to Ethiopia and saw the plight of the fistula women. 'Fistula pilgrims', Reg called them, on account of the formidable journeys they made to seek help. Since then the hospital has restored more than 32,000 from wretched despair to joyous new life.

Reg died in 1993 but Catherine carries on, and at an age when most women are content just to reflect upon their memories, she is working as hard as ever. She is intimately involved with every aspect of the hospital, still doing rounds, still operating.

At the nurses' station inside the ward she consults her colleagues about tomorrow's list. There are seven cases of varying degrees of difficulty. She pores over the notes, contained in green cardboard folders. They give a brief history of the patient – how many days she was in labour, where she came from, how she got here, how many previous children she has borne, any medical information that will affect her management. The doctor who did the initial examination has drawn a diagram showing the location and size of the fistula. Catherine chooses her cases. Let us meet one of them.

Amina Mohamed is twenty, a heart-stopping beauty with glowing black skin, finely sculpted features, and wide, limpid eyes revealing an alert intelligence. Amina comes from the eastern part of Ethiopia, where the land rises in a series of jagged ridges from the Awash River to over 2000 metres. Impossible country, this, for motor vehicles. If you need to travel, you go on foot, ride a donkey, or if you fall ill, must be carried on a litter made of poles and goatskin. It will be many hours, maybe days, before you reach a road, never mind a hospital.

In a developed country Amina would have the world at her feet. But here her future is ordained from birth. Marriage. Children. Work. Death. Eternity. Motherhood is the most important thing to her. Without children she is nothing.

When she was ten her father arranged her marriage to a boy from a neighbouring village; her worth – two goats and a cow. When the deal was done her parents informed her that she was engaged, which was kind of them; often a bride does not even know she is to be married until her wedding day.

At fourteen she was judged old enough to become a wife. On her wedding day her husband's parents held a celebration at their home. *Injera* was served, a kind of rubbery pancake which is the staple of Ethiopia, and a special *wat* (stew) of goat in honour of the occasion. The men beat drums and danced. The women looked on, wailing an unearthly ululation that signified approval. Amina waited alone in her parent's *tukul*, nervous about what was shortly to happen.

After many hours the wedding party made their way to her

village. Her father led her outside to meet her new husband. Hesitantly, she mounted the donkey he had brought, then, glancing wistfully back now and again, set off for her new home.

Like many Ethiopian children Amina was stunted due to her poor diet. At fourteen she had not yet had her first period. Her husband obeyed his parents' instructions not to touch his bride until she was a woman. In the meantime she did her chores, fetching water and firewood, grinding the grain for *injera*. She learnt the ways of the household and got to know her husband a little better. She missed her family. She was sometimes frightened at the thought of being a proper wife and having children, but comforted herself with the knowledge that she would only be doing what millions of other women had done.

At fifteen her childhood ended. Three years later she fell pregnant.

The first labour pains came in the middle of the night. She did not wake her husband as he had to rise early to work the fields. This was women's business. By dawn the contractions were coming at regular intervals. Her mother-in-law helped her from the straw mattress on its earthen platform at one side of the *tukul*, onto the floor. Her mother arrived a couple of hours later to assist. With the two women supporting her, one on either side, Amina squatted all that day, pushing and pushing, wracked by regular waves of pain.

By the time night fell the baby had not yet been born. Amina was very tired. She lay down on the mattress; sleep was impossible.

The contractions continued all that night and into the following day without any sign of the baby emerging. The two older women encouraged Amina to continue pushing, but by now she was so exhausted that she could no longer keep squatting. She lay on the mattress whimpering with pain, occasionally steeling herself to get up and try again. *Please let the baby come. Why doesn't it come?*

Another night. As the sun stole into the valley next day with still no change, Amina knew that something was terribly wrong. She had no idea what to do except to summon all of her will to push and push against the pain. All that day, for hour after weary hour, the contractions continued. The older women knew that the baby must be dead. It was the mother's life that they feared for now.

That night when her husband came home from the fields the family discussed what to do. At dawn the following day, the third after her labour had begun, two of Amina's cousins helped her to her feet and led her gently to the pathway out of the village. She staggered forwards, pausing for support each time the contractions struck. One hour passed. Two. Slowly they made their way up and down the steep hills, every step a trial of endurance. After more than three hours they reached the road which led to the regional capital, Harar.

The cousins flagged down a truck. While the driver revved his engine impatiently, they lifted Amina onto the tray. For an hour and a half they bumped along the gravel road. Amina, drifting in and out of consciousness, was delirious with pain.

There is a small hospital in Harar but there was no one there who was qualified to perform a caesarean section. The outpatients nurse told the cousins that they would have to take Amina to Nazareth, a further 60 kilometres away. This time they caught the bus, arriving at the hospital in the early evening. This hospital was set up for emergency obstetrics. Later that night Amina gave herself up to the heavenly oblivion of anaesthetic. The doctor made a swift incision. The baby, of course, was long dead.

When Amina woke in the morning she was tired and weak, and her abdomen hurt where she had been cut. She looked about her, taking in the other beds in the ward, some people leaning over a patient, a nurse writing on a clipboard. Gradually she became aware that something was not right. It took her a few moments to realise with dismay that the bed was saturated. She rose and shakily made her way to the washroom. She cleaned herself as best she could, but what was this? Her bodily wastes continued to leak, trickling down her legs onto the floor. The odour was terrible.

The hospital could not wait to get rid of Amina. She was discharged that same day, to make her way back over rough roads and winding pathways to her home. As daylight faded she made excuses to remain outside the *tukul* for as long as she could. She only nibbled at a tiny bit of food, and drank as little as possible. Before finally going indoors to sleep, she washed herself once more. That night when she lay down beside her husband, she kept perfectly still with her legs closed tightly together. In the middle of the night she was woken by her husband shaking her. Her clothing and the mattress were dirty. The smell was overpowering. Roughly he pushed her off the platform and ordered her to sleep on the floor.

Amina did not want her husband to see her like this. The next day she returned to her parents, thinking that she would stay there until whatever had broken inside her had healed. She went to the village well once but the other women turned away holding their noses, and one or two taunted her cruelly. After a few days even her parents could not bear to have her in their living quarters. She moved into a broken-down little hut which had been used to house farming implements. There she passed her time, dejected and alone.

So far this had been a typical Ethiopian tale – one that usually ends with a lifetime of misery for the woman involved. But someone in the village had heard of a place in the capital, Addis Ababa, where it was said that women with Amina's complaint could be cured. And, as unbelievable as it might sound, the treatment was free.

At first Amina's husband visited her now and then, but his appearances became less and less frequent. Four months had passed when, during one of these visits, Amina asked if he would give her the money to travel to the capital. He refused. He told Amina that she was of no use to him in this condition. He had wasted enough time on her and certainly wasn't going to waste more money. He was divorcing her.

Amina's parents loved their daughter. Although they were desperately poor, her father found the money for her bus fare to the capital. He did not feel he could take her himself as he knew nothing of cities and did not speak the language. A cousin was again called upon to help.

I can only guess at Amina's embarrassment at being in public in her state, or her dejection when bus drivers refused to allow her on board, or the undisguised disgust of the passengers who were eventually persuaded to endure her presence. I first met Amina when she arrived at the gate of the Fistula Hospital, humiliated and weeping. The guard directed her towards the outpatients department. As she made her way down the drive-way and across the stone-flagged forecourt, she must have felt she had entered another world: of clean white buildings, well-kept lawns and flower gardens ablaze with colour. The admissions staff welcomed her kindly. She was examined by a doctor in a white coat who told her that they would help her. She was bathed, given a clean gown and a gaily coloured woollen shawl, and assigned a bed in one of the wards, along with dozens of other women who were awaiting surgery.

Now there is a third character to meet – the storyteller. In the year 2000 I came to the hospital to help Dr Catherine Hamlin write her biography. A biographer is a dilettante. You invade someone's life, questioning them, their friends and family, and sometimes their enemies. You peck out your few thousand words and you move on. Or sometimes not. The achievements of some people are so remarkable that even after the book has been published, you feel you have barely begun to tell the story. Catherine Hamlin was one of these. She is a marvel. The *New York Times* said of her, 'Dr Hamlin is the new Mother Teresa of our age.' The institution which Catherine and Reg founded has spawned stories to fill several books. So here I am seven years later, living in the compound once more, observing Catherine at work, meeting the other doctors who are devoted to her cause, and hearing patients' stories – tales of heartbreak and triumph that make you weep and rejoice by turns. So many stories . . . so many transformed lives.

CHAPTER 1

At eight o'clock in the morning Amina is wheeled into the theatre. She is helped onto the operating table, where she sits with her legs dangling. Her gown is undone at the back and she is instructed to lean forward. A nurse standing in front of her cradles her head against her chest, murmuring words of reassurance. To the onlooker it's a strangely tender little tableau. Trust and compassion embodied in one poignant moment. The anaesthetist administers a spinal injection, an epidural, to make Amina numb from the waist down. The anaesthetic will last for about two hours. If the operation goes on longer and she begins to feel pain they can keep going with morphine for another fifteen minutes. After that there is another drug, Ketamine, they can use. Most operations take less than two hours.

Amina lies on her back and her feet are placed in stirrups. There are three tables in this big, open room, all within sight of each other. Another operation is already under way and Amina can see the green-gowned staff grouped around the patient, the flash of stainless-steel instruments. What must she be thinking, having come from a rural peasant existence to this? Amina's lower body is draped with green cloths until only her vagina is revealed. The

11

bed is tilted so that her head is pointing slightly downhill. When all is ready Catherine sits on a stool at the foot of the table.

Protocol dictates that she is never addressed as Catherine; it's always Dr Hamlin. The theatre nurse stands on her right side with the instrument tray, and an assistant surgeon stands at her left.

Catherine is feeling a little off colour today. She has spent the past few days in bed with amoebic dysentery. A doctor would advise her not to work, but here she *is* the doctor, and there is no question of her taking the day off. 'If I collapse, Dr Haile can take over,' she says brightly. Dr Hailegiorgis is one of the senior surgeons.

Catherine has lost count of the number of fistula operations she has done. She and Reg together did about 6000 in the sixteen years they were at a government-run hospital; they probably did 500 a year in the first few years at the Fistula Hospital before other doctors arrived to take some of the load. She still loves surgery and she sees no reason to stop just because she's 83. 'It keeps me going,' she says.

She believes that most surgeons retire earlier than they need to. The only reason to stop is if your hands start shaking and hers are still as steady as a girl's. Her eyesight is excellent. She wears spectacles only for distance.

When the Hamlins first came to Ethiopia in 1959, they knew nothing about fistulas. Very few doctors in the developed world had ever seen one. Catherine and Reg had been hired by the Ethiopian government on a three-year contract to work in the Princess Tsehai teaching hospital in Addis Ababa. They were to practise obstetrics and gynaecology and found a school of midwifery.

They hadn't been there long before they noticed smelly,

wretched women being turned away from the hospital gate. When they enquired, they were told it was a waste of time even examining them, as their injuries were incurable. After seeing these women's pitiable state and hearing about the hardships they had endured to get there, the Hamlins were determined to try to help.

They began by seeking out whatever information they could about fistula surgery. The earliest recorded fistula had been discovered in the mummified remains of an Egyptian woman who lived around 2050 BC. Fistulas were mentioned in the writings of ancient Hindu medicine, the Vedas and the Upavedas, and the ancient Persians also wrote about them.

From about the seventeenth century, European physicians were recording attempts at repair. One of the difficulties was finding sutures that did not cause infection. A Dutch physician, Hendrick van Roonhuyze, described closing the denuded edges with 'stitching needles made of stiff swan's quills'. Although he recorded two successes, van Roonhuyze believed surgical cure was practically impossible. Over the following centuries gold wire was tried, as was lead. In the mid-1800s a surgeon called Wutzer, in Bonn, cured eleven of 35 cases. One of these, Lucy Stitch, underwent 35 operations until he was successful – and this was long before the discovery of anaesthetics.

In 1834 a British surgeon, Montague Gosset, wrote a letter to *The Lancet* describing the successful use of gold wire, instead of the normal silk or goose quill, for sutures. The advantage, he found, was that there was little ulceration or irritation, yet it had a great ability to keep the edges of the wound together indefinitely.

At about the same time a brilliant American surgeon, John Peter Mettauer of Virginia, operated successfully on at least half a dozen cases using wire sutures twisted together. The cut ends projected just beyond the vulval verge and were sheathed in oiled silk to help stop irritation. They were re-tightened at regular intervals. While the patient was healing, Mettauer used a silver catheter to drain the bladder.

Difficulties included the inaccessible space of the operative area, and the tendency for urine to contaminate the wound while it was healing. Little by little the principles of fistula surgery were discovered. The use of various instruments to aid working in a confined space, catheters to drain the bladder during convalescence, and suture material of non-reactive metal were all important. The problem was that no one was yet able to produce consistent results. It needed someone with a special genius to pull these facets together. That man was an American, Dr James Marion Sims.

Sims was born in 1813 in Lancaster County, South Carolina. After gaining an MD from Jefferson Medical College, he moved to Mount Meigs, Alabama, to practise. The first fistula sufferer he encountered was a seventeen-year-old slave named Anarcha. How familiar her plight sounds today. When Sims saw her, Anarcha had been in labour for three days and her baby was already dead. He pulled out the little corpse with forceps and the girl seemed to be making a recovery. Then, after five days, there was a sudden loss of control of both her bladder and rectum. Sims told Anarcha's employer that her condition was incurable and that he should take care of her for as long as she lived.

Within two months, two more slaves, Betsy and Lucy, had come to him with fistulas, but after examining them he concluded that these too were hopeless. He sent Betsy back to her master and gave Lucy a bed in a little hospital attached to his house while she waited for the next train to take her home.

Like many surgeons before him and many since, Sims became obsessed with the challenge of fistula surgery. One of the most vexing problems was the lack of access to the injured area. Fistula surgery has been described as like operating inside the toe of a shoe. One day Sims had an idea. He bought a pewter spoon then ordered two medical students who were working with him to prepare Lucy for an examination.

Telling her to kneel with her head in her hands, he instructed the students to part the nates (buttocks) and introduced the bent spoon handle into the vagina. Then, as he wrote in his auto-biography, *The Story of My Life*, 'I saw everything as no man had ever seen before. The fistula was as plain as the nose on a man's face. The edges were clear and well defined and distinct . . . I said at once, "Why can not these things be cured?"'

Sims immediately began designing instruments for the opera-tion. The bent spoon was refined to become the Sims speculum – an instrument still used in modified form. He wrote to the owners of Anarcha and Betsy and asked them to send the girls back, and scoured the country for other cases.

When all was ready he operated on Lucy. The procedure failed. Nevertheless, he persevered with his long-suffering and ever-hopeful patients. Gradually, he eliminated one technical problem after another, but still he kept failing. One obstacle remained – he needed some way of tying sutures high up in the body where he could not reach. At three o'clock one morning, lying sleepless in bed, he hit upon the idea of using perforated lead shot which he would slide up the suture and compress with forceps when drawn tight.

In great excitement he again performed the operation on Lucy. He waited a week to see the result. When he examined her it was, as usual, a complete failure.

Sims would not admit defeat. He had improved his operation until it was as near perfect as he could make it, yet still there was something wrong. He wondered if it could be the silk thread he used for sutures. He had heard of earlier surgeons using metal and had tried a leaden suture himself without success. Musing on the problem one day as he was walking from his house to his office, in the yard he picked up a little piece of fine brass wire, which had probably been used as a spring for suspenders. It was as fine as horsehair. He took it to his jeweller and asked him to make some silver wire of the same diameter.

Anarcha was chosen for the experiment. It was the thirtieth time he had operated on her. Stoically she mounted the operating table and prepared to endure once more the probing and cutting without anaesthetic. Sims brought the fistula together with four of his fine silver wires and fixed them with lead shot. As she had done so many times before, Anarcha went to bed to allow the healing process to take place. He waited out the next week in a fever of impatience, then, with a palpitating heart he turned Anarcha on her side, introduced the speculum, 'and there lay the suture apparatus exactly as I had placed it. There was no inflammation, nothing unnatural, and a very perfect union of the fistula.'

Over the next few weeks Lucy and Betsy and all the other patients were cured. Sims was in no doubt about the importance of what he had done. 'I realised the fact that, at last, my efforts had been blessed with success, and that I had made, perhaps, one of the most important discoveries of the age for the relief of suffering humanity.'

Catherine and Reg got a copy of Sims's autobiography from England and sat up late at night avidly reading about his techniques. In 1855 Sims had founded the world's first fistula hospital in New York. Before many years had passed they would build the second.

About a year after Catherine and Reg had arrived in Ethiopia they were ready for their first attempt at fistula surgery. Many of the techniques had improved since Sims's day. For instance, with modern sutures it was no longer necessary to use wire, and instruments were more sophisticated. They chose a relatively easy case – a girl from the provinces with a small hole in her bladder. Reg performed the operation and Catherine assisted. They put her to bed to convalesce and, just as Sims must have so often done, waited anxiously as the days dragged by. She was a brave little girl, trusting and calm. She had no idea that her case was such a landmark for the Hamlins. After about fourteen days they took out the catheter which had been draining her bladder and she was passing urine normally. She went home completely cured.

Nearly five decades and over 30,000 operations later, there is an atmosphere of businesslike calm in the theatre as Catherine draws the lips of Amina's labia aside and secures them with temporary stitches to her inner thighs. A speculum, a modern version of Sims's bent spoon, is inserted to widen the opening. On the face of it, fistula surgery sounds straightforward. You're just closing a hole, right? But the variations and complications are legion. It's not like abdominal surgery, where everything is laid out and open. Everything is hard to get at and difficult to see. New surgeons say that until you've tried it, you just don't realise how hard it is.

Catherine begins to separate the bladder from the surrounding tissue, using scissors which are specially made in England for the hospital. 'Mobilising', they call it. It's done so that there will be no tension on the fistula when they stitch the edges together.

'Sweetheart, this needle is much too big. Give me a smaller one.' Catherine is unfailingly polite when she addresses her colleagues. The nurses are all 'sweetheart' or 'darling'.

The nurse hands her a tiny, curved needle already threaded. Catherine grasps it in a complicated-looking holder and manoeuvres it deftly into the restricted space. She passes it through flesh and through again, ties the stitch and holds the free ends for her assistant to snip off.

Her assistant today is Mamitu, although Catherine always calls her by the pet name Mamite (Mameet). Of all the stories from the hospital hers is one of the most compelling. She was once a patient herself – an illiterate peasant girl of sixteen who was carried in to the old Princess Tsehai Hospital in 1962, close to death. She had already been badly injured after enduring four days of labour. Further horrific damage was done when the *wogesha*, an untrained village 'doctor', cut her with a blunt old knife and dragged the dead baby out by brute force.

Over the years, Mamitu endured operation after operation. But her injuries were so severe that it was impossible to make her whole again. She could never return to normal life in her village, so the Hamlins gave her work to do and a permanent place to live in the hospital. At first she helped make beds in the ward. She graduated to theatre duties and eventually ended up assisting Reg. To begin with she'd just hand him instruments or tie off a stitch or two, but she was so naturally gifted that she became more and more involved in the actual surgery. She is now a skilled fistula surgeon.

Catherine asks Mamitu to insert catheters into the tiny openings in the ureters, the two narrow tubes that run from the kidneys to the bladder. They are so hard to see that it's easy to stitch one accidentally. The catheters make them more visible. Because of their size, the ureters are difficult to locate, especially when the anatomy has been distorted by scar tissue. Whenever Reg or Catherine had trouble they always used to call upon Mamitu. Asked how she does it, she replies, 'I just pray to God.'

The hole in the rectum is an easy one, according to Catherine. Only small. The one in the bladder is quite big, but because Amina has come to them soon after the birth there's none of the scarring that always makes the repair more difficult.

Three-quarters of an hour into the operation Amina calls out in distress. The anaesthetist has been monitoring her but with everyone else clustered around the foot of the table you almost forget that there's a real person under those drapes. She begins to cry. Her head is hurting. The anaesthetist comforts her with a few soft words, and she settles down, staring fixedly at the ceiling.

Some surgeons like to chat, even crack jokes when they work. Catherine and Mamitu don't say much, beyond what is necessary for the task at hand. They've been working together for so long that they hardly need to speak. If the incision needs to be swabbed, or Catherine needs an instrument to be held in a certain position, or help with an especially tricky suture, it's done before she asks for it.

It's an hour and a half into the procedure. Catherine ties off the final stitch. Now comes a critical moment, when they will see if the repair is watertight. The nurse injects some purple-coloured liquid through a catheter into the bladder. If there is a leak the dye will reveal it. They wait in silence for a few moments. No sign of purple. The repair is good. Catherine dabs some gentian violet on the wound. 'This hides all our sins,' she quips.

Closing the hole isn't the end of the story, though. About 92 per cent of these operations are successful. But sometimes the repair breaks down and has to be done again. And of that 92 per cent of patients, maybe 30 per cent will suffer from incontinence because of other damage. Amina will have to wait a couple of weeks before they can say that she is cured.

They take her legs out of the stirrups, tie her gown, and wheel her away to the recovery ward. Usually Catherine would do another operation or two, visit patients, attend meetings, write letters or e-mails. But the concentrated effort has taken its toll and she's ready to go back to bed to try to fight off that persistent amoeba once and for all.

CHAPTER 2

In their first few years Catherine and Reg were able to fit in the fistula surgery around their other work at the government hospital. As word of their success spread, more and more patients began arriving from all over Ethiopia. One woman walked 450 kilometres from the north of the country to Addis Ababa. Another, from down near the Kenyan border, had begged at the bus stop for seven years to raise the fare to the capital. Reg used to drive his Volkswagen Beetle down to the bus station every day and ask around for anyone smelling of urine. He'd round up a group of patients, pile them into the car and take them back to the hospital. His eight-year-old son, Richard, once asked his father, 'Daddy, why do we always have to have the car smelling of urine?' In the outpatients department the other women would push the fistula pilgrims down to the end of the queue because of the smell. Reg would put his arms around them and say, 'You're the most important patient here today, so you can go to the front.'

There was nowhere to put the women while they waited for surgery, so the Hamlins bedded them down in storerooms, underneath stairwells – anywhere they could find space. It soon became obvious that they needed a proper place. In 1962, three years after they'd arrived in Ethiopia, Catherine and Reg built a hostel with ten beds to house waiting patients. Almost immediately they found that it was not big enough, and it was later expanded to 30 beds. Often it was so crowded that the women were sleeping two to a bed.

By the end of the 1960s the fistula patients were taking up an enormous amount of the Hamlins' time and stretching the hospital's resources to breaking point. It was obvious that something had to be done. In 1971, using money donated from New Zealand, they bought a piece of land on the outskirts of the city beside a pretty little river. Four years later, in 1975, they opened the hospital, devoted solely to fistula surgery.

From the beginning they set world's best practice standards of patient care and hygiene. Visiting doctors from other hospitals in Ethiopia would just shake their heads in envy and amazement. As the number of patients grew, the hospital steadily expanded. Every three years, under their contract with the Ethiopian government, Reg and Catherine would take overseas leave. They would use some of the time away to raise money, mainly in America and Australia. 'We were always begging,' says Catherine. And the donations always seemed to arrive just when some new piece of equipment was needed, or another building, or some more staff salaries.

In 1993 Reg died from cancer. He was 85, fourteen years older than Catherine. At first Catherine did not believe that she'd be able to carry on by herself. They had done everything together and Reg had taken most of the burden of fund-raising and administration. One morning, not long after Reg died, she went out at dawn to sit on her verandah and pray. She was overwhelmed by the feeling that everything was too much for her. A storeman, Birru, who had been with the Hamlins since he was a teenager, appeared. He knelt beside her, took her hand and kissed it. 'Don't leave us,' he said. 'We'll all help you.'

Catherine was so touched that she wept. Birru's words and actions were just what she had needed. She pushed aside any thought of not carrying on. As she wrote in *The Hospital by the River*, 'I began to realise the enormous blessings that I had, and the future seemed suddenly bright and exciting.'

One of the key people at the hospital is Sister Ruth Kennedy. Ruth, a medical missionary, came to the hospital in the year 2000 to handle the increasing amount of public relations work required. Her story is worth a book in itself. She was brought up in Brazil, the child of missionary parents who lived and worked in the pitifully poor *favellas* (slums) of the capital, São Paulo.

She remembers her mother bringing home the neglected children of prostitutes and finding homes for them. Her father founded churches; one of them serviced a community who lived in the municipal rubbish dump scavenging refuse for a living. Ruth studied midwifery and did a course at an American Bible college, and at the age of 29 went to the poorest nation on earth, Chad, to work in a mission hospital. Almost immediately she caught malaria, and after six months she came down with hepatitis. During the times she was well enough, she worked practically around the clock as a midwife, dealing with women who were often on the verge of death.

'Women would come in on ox carts, completely septic with a retained placenta or ruptured uterus. If the babies were dead already I never felt it so badly, but some of them had a live baby resting between their breasts. It was the little live babies cuddled up against this dead body that affected me. If you didn't catch them in time, the relatives would bury the baby with the mother. So I would rescue these little babies. When they realised I would take them they stopped burying them and brought them to me instead.'

Ruth remembers looking after three babies at once, bottle-feeding them in her double bed. When they were strong enough she would take the babies to a Swiss couple who ran a children's home. They found adoptive parents for them locally and in Europe. After she'd been there a year, civil war broke out between two tribes, the Zaghawa and the Goran. Ruth was conducting Bible studies with local women early in the morning before they went to the market. Some of them were killed on their way to attend the class; their deaths had nothing to do with religion, they just happened to belong to the wrong tribe. Ruth decided that it was time to leave.

Ruth went to England for a while, and when the war ended, returned to Chad to work for another mission hospital. She set up a team which went into the villages teaching men and women primary health – how to deal with malaria and diarrhoea, burns and cuts, safe delivery of babies and so on. She stayed in Chad for the next ten years, until she felt that God was calling her to go to Ethiopia.

She came to Ethiopia with a one-month visa, took a twelve-month lease on a house in Addis Ababa and went looking for a job. In the waiting room at the British Embassy one day she sat next to a nun, who, in a thick Irish accent, asked Ruth, 'You're not a midwife, are you?'

'I am.'

'You don't teach, do you?'

'I do.'

'Good, we need you.'

The nun gave her a contact in the Ministry of Health. There she was told once again, 'We need you.' But, as is the way in Ethiopia, there was a tortuous bureaucratic maze to negotiate before the need could be met. While Ruth was filling in forms and endlessly waiting in government offices, she renewed her visa three times, and at one stage had to leave the country to spend some time in England. From there she wrote a letter to the Fistula Hospital asking for a job. She teases Catherine about it now. 'You didn't want me here,' she tells her.

'Never, that's not true.'

But the proof is there, a letter of rejection written in Catherine's own hand.

Back in Addis, Ruth started going to language school. Sometimes she'd come and visit the Fistula Hospital to practise. During these visits she and Catherine got to know one another. With their medical backgrounds and shared Christian faith, they had plenty in common, and Ruth's compassion for the poor and dispossessed of this world was something Catherine could well relate to.

In 1994 Ruth was finally registered as a midwife and went to teach at a new school which had opened in Harar. She'd been there about three months when some young men from a local church came to see her with a baby they'd found abandoned. They'd been out walking by the city walls when they saw hyenas gathered around something on the ground. They thought they'd have a bit of fun chasing them away. When they did they heard a mewling sound. It was a baby boy, so new that he still had the umbilical cord attached. Ruth took the child in and looked after him. Word soon got around that the *ferenji* (foreigner) would accept orphaned babies. Over the next two and a half years she took in fifteen, caring for them until homes could be found.

The only one they couldn't find a place for was a little boy, Masrasha. His mother had contracted AIDS after being gang-raped. She was pregnant when Ruth met her. When the baby was born Ruth showed her how to care for him. The mother wanted to put him up for adoption, so they tested him and found he had AIDS as well. Ruth took him to the Mother Teresa home, The Missionaries of Charity. They took him in and at the age of two months he died. His mother died two years later.

Ruth got involved with counselling girls who had HIV/AIDS. The girls would come into Harar from the country to work in the bars. Once they got used to the environment they'd be given to the men. She'll never forget some of their stories. 'There was one beautiful little girl who got AIDS, and she didn't have anyone, so I cared for her at my house. I remember one time I said, "What would you like to eat?"

'She said, "Do you think you could buy me sardines?"

'"Yes, I could buy you sardines."

'She ate one. She said they just go down easier. She died two days later. Funny the things you remember about people, isn't it? She just wanted sardines.

'There was another little girl who said, "Would you be like my mother?"

'I told her, "Sure, I could be like your mother."

'She said, "You know, I don't know what's happened to me." You could see the ravages of AIDS. This was before the western nations had decided that Africa was worth anything, so that we could have the anti-retroviral treatment. There was nothing at that time, so these little girls would just die with all these dreadful diseases, Kaposi's sarcoma, diarrhoea . . . they'd waste away before your eyes. There wasn't anything you could do for them. My little sardine girl, as I called her, was seventeen.'

Harar is an old walled city which is predominantly Muslim. In 1996 a woman friend of Ruth's who was working for the Danish mission was killed by extremists. She had her nose and ears cut off. Ruth took it as a sign that it was probably time to move on.

Her next job was with the Ministry of Health, training nurses all over the country in emergency obstetrics. It was valuable experience for her later work at the Fistula Hospital. She made many government contacts and gained an intimate knowledge of how the bureaucracy works.

Early in Ruth's stay at Harar, Catherine had asked her to become a trustee of the hospital. From regular attendance at trustee meetings she learnt how the place worked. That, coupled with her medical background and her intimate knowledge of the Ethiopian bureaucracy, made her an invaluable acquisition. At dinner one night a trustee, Geoffrey Weatherill, asked if she would consider coming to work there. Ruth said, 'Just let me finish my time at the Ministry of Health and I'll come.' She arrived in January 2000 to take up the job of public relations officer.

Ruth is a doer. I go to her office, a little round building with a conical roof, like a modern version of a village *tukul*, to ask about a patient whose progress I've been following.

'We'll go find her,' she says. She grabs a handful of little bottles of makeup which an American visitor has left, and strides out of the office towards the outpatients department. Ruth is a big-boned woman with a no-nonsense manner. There's the usual group of women outside the outpatients: a few patients in their hospital gowns and shawls, mixed with peasant women in travel-stained *gabis*, newly arrived from the country. Ruth sweeps up to one of them who's waiting patiently on a bench to see a doctor, launches into a stream of Amharic and gives her a bottle before moving off. The woman looks at it in bewilderment without saying a word.

Seeing a patient she knows, Ruth envelops her in a hug. Ethiopians are small people and this little lady practically disappears in her embrace. Ruth speaks to her for a few moments in a torrent of Amharic, bursts into loud laughter, which gets a shy smile in return, then off Ruth goes again into the ward.

In a bed near the entrance she spies one of the nurse aides from the new fistula hospital at Bahar Dar in northern Ethiopia, who has been sent down to recover from a complex operation. Ruth whips out her mobile phone, speed-dials Bahar Dar and as soon as she gets an answer hands the phone to the patient.

After chatting to her colleague for a minute or two, the patient hands it back with a big smile. While she has been speaking Ruth has handed out the rest of the makeup bottles to half a dozen bemused patients. A couple of them clearly have no idea what they are, so she undoes the bottle and demonstrates the makeup to them.

The girl we are seeking is discovered to be in another ward, so off we go again, marching purposefully through the grounds, Ruth talking over her shoulder as I hurry to keep up. In the other ward we find our patient sitting up in bed sewing. Ruth strides over to her and gives her a big hug. 'Come on, let's show how we can dance!' she cries.

Grinning, the girl, Tanashe, gets out of bed. Ruth sets the rhythm with clapping hands and Tanashe starts to dance. A crowd of other patients gathers, smiling broadly, and soon they are all dancing and laughing, Ruth included. She carries her own energy field along with her and the girls love her for it.

There are two main things that drive Ruth Kennedy: her love of God and her love of Catherine Hamlin. In some ways she has filled the space left by Reg's death. She is Catherine's confidante and adviser. Whenever Catherine travels abroad, Ruth goes with her. Together they make many of the day-to-day decisions affecting the hospital.

They know one another as well as a married couple would. At a dinner party one night at Ruth's house within the compound, she goes to the kitchen to bring in the food. Catherine calls out,

'Do you need any help, Ruth?' Then, in an aside to the others at the table, 'I'm quite safe in asking. I always ask and she always says no.'

On cue from the kitchen comes Ruth's reply, 'No thanks.'

When the meal, which, as with all meals involving Catherine, has been accompanied by plenty of good talk and laughter, ends, Ruth goes back to the kitchen.

'Need any help, Ruth?' asks Catherine.

In unison everyone at the table joins in Ruth's reply, 'No thanks,' then we all break up with laughter.

Later there is another little routine which feels familiar. Ruth places on the table a wooden case with felted compartments, each containing a different type of tea. One of them is the African herbal tea, Rooibos. Catherine dislikes Rooibos and furthermore, can never pronounce its name properly. She calls it Robot. Ruth knows this very well. 'Catherine, would you like some Rooibos?' she enquires, with just the hint of a smile.

'No. You know I can't stand Robot.'

There follows a discussion of the merits of various teas. Each time Catherine mentions Robot, the table breaks up. It is all very innocent, and old-fashioned and charming.

From about the time that Ruth arrived, great changes began to occur at the hospital. After decades of the Hamlins living hand to mouth, constantly begging for funds, important bodies such as the United Nations, the World Health Organization, USAID and others, began to take an interest in the plight of fistula sufferers in the developing world. The resulting influx of funds has brought with it many benefits but also new problems. All great institutions have critical moments in their evolution. While it is still pre-eminent, Reg and Catherine's little hospital no longer has the field to itself. There are now other organisations competing for those funds. How Catherine, Ruth and the other key people involved in decision-making for the hospital handle the challenge of rapid expansion will be crucial to its future success.

CHAPTER 3

In the early days Reg used to take each patient aside after she'd been admitted and explain what had caused her injury. He'd tear a hole in a piece of paper, leaving the flap still attached, and pour on some water so that it drained through the hole. He'd close the flap and explain that that was what they were going to do in the operating theatre. If their husband or relatives were there he'd include them in the discussion as well.

These days Reg's simple demonstration has been replaced by a professionally made video. It's shown several times a day in a section of the outpatients department which has benches to accommodate about twenty viewers. Actors play out a scene familiar to every woman who comes here – the long, agonising labour; a dead baby; humiliation and rejection; the arduous trip to the hospital; the operation; and at the end – a new life for the patient.

Today there are about ten women and one or two men watching. Some of the women have already been in the hospital for a while, but still come to see the video time and time again, as if for reassurance that the miracle they long for is really possible.

★

A woman arrives wearing a grey-coloured *gabi* and carrying a yellow plastic bag containing all her belongings. These *gabis* start out white, but quickly become so soiled that no amount of washing them in a cold mountain stream will restore them. She's alone. She looks tired, and a bit frightened. In the reception area the nurse in charge of outpatients, Sister Konjit, welcomes her with a smile and passes her over to the admissions clerk, Negussi, who takes down her particulars.

I ask Konjit if she will translate for me. The woman's name is Alganish. She comes from halfway between Gonder and Tigray, way up in the northern part of Ethiopia. She has been travelling for two days to get here. Alganish has five living children. Three were her first husband's. He died six years ago. She remarried and had two more. Four months ago she had a long, difficult labour which ended with the baby being stillborn.

One of her brothers walked for two days to reach her village, then he and some other male family members carried her for a day to reach the road. After that she went by car to the new fistula hospital at Mekele. She says she was terribly embarrassed riding in the car because of the way she smelled, and the seat got wet. Her injuries were too serious to be treated at Mekele, so they gave her the money to go to Addis Ababa. Because of her condition the trip was very difficult, she says. She was afraid to sleep in a bed in a hotel, so she just slept outside on the ground. She had never been to Addis and was worried that she wouldn't be able to find the hospital. She speaks a little bit of Amharic as well as Tigrinian, so she was able to ask at the bus station.

Alganish tells her story in a matter-of-fact way, without any sign of self-pity. When I ask her how she felt when she had to go out in public she is puzzled. Konjit has to explain the question to her. No one has ever asked her how she feels. She cannot grasp the idea that anyone would care about her emotions.

Her main worry is not for herself, but for her children from her first marriage. They're always fighting with their stepfather and she's concerned that he won't look after them properly while she's away. She joins the other women sitting on benches watching the video while they wait to be examined. Ethiopian women seem to be able to sit quite still for hours on end, waiting passively for whatever is going to befall them. She seems perfectly composed – perhaps her composure is born of fatalism.

A little later another woman arrives, also carrying a yellow plastic bag. You see them everywhere, these bags. Half the women who come to the hospital seem to have them. There's a man with her wearing a shabby jacket, threadbare shirt and pants and broken-down shoes with no socks.

The woman's name is Leteabazgi and she's also from Tigray in the north. She's unable to look at me, and speaks in a tiny little voice. She seems traumatised. Under Sister Konjit's patient questioning her story emerges. She's 23 years old and had her baby four years ago – her first. Her husband left her and she's been living with her mother and father in a one-room hut, afraid to go outside because of her shameful condition. Three years ago she was examined in the general hospital at Adigrat. They told her about the Fistula Hospital but she had no one to bring her here.

The man with her is a soldier. He lives in Addis Ababa but was born in her village and they knew each other growing up. He went back there to attend his sister's funeral. Leteabazgi pleaded with him to take her to Addis. They've been on the road for four days. She only had a little money – not enough to pay for the bus fares and hotels. He didn't have much either, so he suggested she beg from the passengers on the bus. People felt sorry for her, he says, and gave money. He used some of it to buy plastic to put on the seat and on the bed in the hotel. They'd arrived in Addis a day ago and spent the night at his home.

I tell him he's a good man.

'I just want to help for the love of God,' he says.

Leteabazgi is examined by Dr Abiy, a resident who is doing postgraduate study in O&G (obstetrics and gynaecology). Every student who wants to specialise in women's medicine has to spend two months at the Fistula Hospital.

He tells me that Leteabazgi has a vesico-vaginal fistula, which means a hole in the bladder. Because it's taken so long for her to come to the hospital there's a lot of scarring. Also her urethra is very short, not more than 1.5 centimetres. It should be 3 or 4 centimetres. Her bladder is also very small. Because of these factors the outcome may not be good. He means that even if the fistula is cured, she may still suffer from incontinence – stress incontinence, they call it. 'For me the operation would be very difficult,' says Abiy. 'But maybe not for someone who is more experienced.'

He lays it all out for Leteabazgi, and oddly enough she smiles and looks happy for the first time since she arrived. Maybe just knowing that someone is going to try to help makes a difference.

I say to Abiy that she's got a pretty rough few weeks ahead of her, but it will be better than being in her condition without treatment in a hut in a remote village.

He agrees. 'Yes, it's better.'

A few days later Catherine has recovered from her illness and is back in the theatre. This time her assistant is another young resident, Amha. He and Abiy are from Jimma medical school in the south, one of five medical schools in Ethiopia. In fact, Amha and Abiy are room-mates. Catherine has a high opinion of students from Jimma. They are almost always impressive – more so than those from the Black Lion Hospital in Addis. Some of the teachers there are themselves barely a year out of medical school.

Amha's movements are firm and confident. When he has to thread one of the tiny needles he does it perfectly on his first attempt. 'Good boy,' says Catherine. 'I think you must darn your own socks.' All university courses in Ethiopia are taught in English, so Amha is fluent in it.

The hospital is expanding so rapidly that Catherine is worried they won't have enough surgeons in the future. She's always on the lookout for promising talent to recruit. It's not easy to persuade young doctors to devote their lives to fistula surgery. The surgeons at the Fistula Hospital do a small amount of private practice, but doing it full time would be far more lucrative. Many graduates can't wait to leave Ethiopia and seek their fortune in the west. She tells the residents that the real satisfaction of this work is in the results. 'They may not be particularly interested in the surgery but I always say to these boys, just start with small pinholes and you'll get a tremendous joy when the woman is cured. Then you'll be hooked and you'll be able to continue and do bigger cases. Don't start with anything bad. If you have one failure to begin with, that'll be the end of you.'

Catherine tries to assign the young residents straightforward cases, but the trouble is that sometimes you don't realise how difficult a case is until you start operating. At the next table Dr Abiy is operating on a patient named Zemebech. She's from Wollo province in the north-east. She's had six babies, three of whom are alive. The last one was stillborn after three days of labour, leaving her with a fistula. She and her husband are farmers. If there are existing children, the husbands will often stay with their wives; Zemebech left the three children at home with him while her neighbours carried her on a litter to the road. Then she came by bus to Addis Ababa.

In her bladder Zemebech has two big holes which Abiy has

made into one. Where Catherine's movements were swift and decisive, he's fumbling a bit, and taking time to think about what he's going to do next. Mamitu is his assistant. As well as being an excellent surgeon, she is a gifted teacher. In spite of her accomplishments, she has never lost the natural grace and modesty of her peasant upbringing, and her students respond to this. Abiy often goes to drink coffee in the little flat where Mamitu lives in the hospital compound. He's 27, she's 61; yet, they've become good friends. He is a little bit in awe of Mamitu. Maybe there's even a bit of hero-worship going on.

Catherine finishes up her case and comes over to see how Abiy's doing. He grasps a piece of anatomy in the forceps and turns it this way and that, pondering.

'Just cut it off,' says Catherine.

Snip, and into the little bin between his feet it goes. Abiy has impressed Catherine. She's asked him to consider fistula surgery as a career. He's thinking about it, but this experience may not be helping her cause.

Catherine makes some suggestions about how to proceed, and half an hour later Abiy has finished. A nurse injects the dye and they wait a little tensely. Mamitu has a trick that she plays on all her students. When they're not looking she puts a dab of dye onto some gauze, swabs the wound then shows it to the student with a suitably sympathetic look. She could count on an especially good reaction today, after such a difficult procedure, but unfortunately she's already caught Abiy out once. They study the repair. It's good.

At the third table one of the senior surgeons, Dr Biruk, is working on a patient from Somalia. Halema's notes are pretty sketchy, as she speaks only Somali. From what they can gather, she's 35 years old. She was married at eighteen yet only had her first baby a year ago. This is very unusual, as most women have had several children by that age. Biruk thinks she must have had a history of infertility. After a prolonged labour she was left with a dead baby and a fistula. And, to make her story even more tragic, her husband had died when she was four months pregnant. No one in Somalia does fistula surgery. Halema lives in a war zone so it couldn't have been easy to get here.

Biruk is a handsome fellow, a bit of a charmer – tall, fine-featured, with a natty moustache and a sharp sense of humour. There's a lot of giggling going on between him and the nurses. He likes to give his assistants nicknames. For instance he used to call today's 'Sara Ampol', which is the name of a high-tech theatre light, on account of her excellent eyesight. Today she's apparently been a bit below par; she's missed threading a couple of needles, so he's renamed her 'the candle'. 'I don't mean it,' he says. 'I'm just teasing her. She's excellent.'

Biruk reckons it's important to be a bit lighthearted now and then. 'When things are complicated with surgeons it's sometimes very quiet. Sometimes we shout too. If there's no complications we have a bit of a joke now and then.'

Biruk repairs Halema's fistula but suspects she's also suffering from stress incontinence, because relative to the size of the hole there was a lot of leakage, so he does a correctional procedure to the urethra. He's not at all confident that she'll be cured.

Throughout the hour and three-quarters of the operation, Halema lies quiet and uncomplaining. As they release her feet from the stirrups and tie her gown she leans over and vomits neatly onto the floor.

One of the newer surgeons, Dr Habte, is operating on a 26-year-old woman named Letelibanes. She has a son aged six. Three years ago her second child was stillborn, after three days of labour. There's no joking with Dr Habte. He works with pain-staking care and an air of great seriousness. I'm never sure in an operating theatre whether it's okay just to butt in and start asking questions. I hesitate for a few minutes, then choose a moment when he seems to be taking a pause. He's happy to explain his case.

When he saw Letelibanes in outpatients, Dr Habte thought that it was going to be a difficult operation. But now that she's on the table under anaesthetic, it's not as difficult as he expected. He's confident about closing the fistula, but there are some other factors that may go against a total cure. Like Leteabazgi, she has a short urethra and her bladder size is small, so she may still have stress incontinence even after the fistula has been repaired.

And so it goes. Habte finishes his procedure, Mamitu does an operation, Biruk a second one and Catherine another. Seven in all. I am curious to know more about these women: Zemebech, Halema and Letelibanes. Who are they? What have they been through before coming to this place? What have they yet to endure? This morning they were names written in the notes. Now they're people.

After we wrote about Mamitu in *The Hospital by the River* she became something of a celebrity. Someone else has since written a whole book about her, and she was approached by an Italian film producer who wanted to make a movie about her life. She turned down the offer, and now whenever some journalist turns up wanting to write her story, she politely declines.

She has used her salary, plus some money that Reg left her, to buy a little house for her sister, and to educate her nephew, Daniel. Daniel is now the head driver at the hospital and is in charge of maintaining all the vehicles. Mamitu still lives in a little flat in the hospital grounds – actually, hardly a flat, it's like two one-room *tukuls* linked together by a short corridor. She used to share it with two other former patients who worked as nurse aides, Letekidane and Likelesh. Letekidane died in 2003; Likelesh is still there.

It has been seven years since I've seen Mamitu. Late one afternoon I knock on her door. She greets me with her usual reserved politeness. I tell her I'm writing another book and ask if we can have a chat. I can see that she really doesn't want to be interviewed again. She vacillates for a moment, but then her innate politeness takes over and she invites me inside. She lives very simply. There's a small table with two chairs, a sideboard, a couch with a low table in front of it, a two-burner cooker sitting on the sink. That's about the sum of her possessions.

She makes the coffee and places the pot on a cane stand to let it settle. While we wait she sits quietly with her hands clasped in front of her. She does not feel the need to fill up the silence as a western hostess would. On the coffee table are three small, rimless cups on a tray. She pours one carefully, almost reverently, and passes it to me. All of her movements are graceful and unhurried. I am reminded of what Catherine once said about her, that everything she does, she does perfectly. For many years, she was in charge of the ward at the weekends and you could always rely on things running smoothly when Mamitu was there.

I sip the strong black brew. 'So, Mamite, how many doctors are here now?'

She ticks them off on her fingers: Dr Ambaye, Dr Mulu, Dr Habte, Dr Haile, Dr Yifru, Dr Biruk and, of course, Mother.

'And you.'

'Oh no. I am not a doctor.'

I ask her about some of the new methods that people are using in fistula surgery. 'Have you changed much since you started?'

'No. I still do the same; but it's good that there are new ways.'

I do not want to interrogate her about her achievements. She's had enough of those questions already. So, instead I remark on how the hospital has expanded since I was last here. 'Is that a good thing?' I wonder.

'Yes, it's a good thing. But it would be better if there were no more fistulas.'

'I think that will be a long time coming.'

'Yes,' she agrees. 'A long time.'

The conversation proceeds at a leisurely pace, as I imagine conversations must have done in the village where Mamitu came from 45 years ago. In some ways she's still that village girl: modest, untroubled by ambition, content with her life. Mamitu has learnt to read and write. She's been going to night school and is now in the fourth grade. Funny, that. The usual thing would be to go to school, then university and then become a world-famous surgeon. But she's doing it the other way around.

CHAPTER 4

Each day at about 8.20 in the morning Catherine makes her way to a large *tukul* that is used as a chapel and a general meeting place. It's called Bete Mesgana, or House of Praise. Anyone who feels like it can come and take part in a brief Bible reading, followed by prayers. Usually about a dozen people turn up, arriving in dribs and drabs, according to the vagaries of the public transport system.

This morning Catherine is there, and Ruth, plus about half a dozen others. The way it works is that Catherine reads the selected passage in English, then one of the Ethiopians reads in Amharic, then two or three people pray in whatever language suits them. The prayers are usually about particular patients or important happenings at the hospital. Today they're praying for one of the nursing sisters, Sister Tsedu. She had been feeling unwell and losing weight for a long time. A month ago one of her colleagues, Sister Methasabeya, convinced her that she should seek medical advice. Doctors found a cancerous mass in her stomach. The Fistula Hospital offered to pay for Tsedu to go to South Africa to see an oncologist, but in the end her sister, who works for Ethiopian Airlines, persuaded her employer to pay for the round trip.

The hospital is covering all of her other expenses.

The reading this morning is from an especially dense passage of Daniel, in the Old Testament. It's hard enough to grasp without an added difficulty – the canine factor. Ruth has recently become mistress of a small, irrepressible puppy of unknown ancestry, named Honey. Whenever anyone opens the door Honey and Catherine's dog, Bunni, who looks like a miniaturised collie, come romping in and start playing about under people's feet. Someone shoos them out and shuts the door, then when the next latecomer turns up, the same thing happens again. Each transgression is received with high good humour by everyone.

After prayers I go back to the little flat where I'm staying. It's a small two-bedroom apartment, which has been built to accommodate visiting doctors from overseas who come to the hospital for training. It overlooks a stone-flagged path which runs from one of the outlying wards to the physiotherapy department underneath the main ward.

Every morning at this time I hear the tap and scrape of patients inching their way along the path using sticks and walking frames. They are women who have been so severely damaged by childbirth that they are sometimes unable to walk at all when they arrive at the hospital. One girl, who looks no more than fifteen, has a dropped foot. This happens when a baby pushing down the birth canal bears so heavily against the nerves leading to the foot that they are damaged. She places her three-pronged walking stick in front of her, steadies, then throws the damaged foot forward by lifting her hip and rotating. Then she drags the other foot forward and repeats the process. Her progress is painful to watch. Behind her comes another girl with a walking frame. I guess her to be about twenty; it's hard to tell ages.

Often when a woman discovers that she's incontinent she will lie still, curled in a foetal position in the hope that she will heal. After weeks – sometimes years – like that, the muscles in her hips and knees and ankles contract, and she can no longer walk.

Sister Azeb is in charge of physiotherapy. She began working as a nurse at the Fistula Hospital ten years ago. She used to help out in the ward with physiotherapy before they had a dedicated unit. When she saw the difference it made, she became more and more interested in it. The hospital noted her enthusiasm and arranged for a succession of physiotherapists from Britain and America to come and train her.

When I go to visit Azeb, there are about a dozen women in the room, shuffling in a line along a long pair of parallel bars under the supervision of a nurse aide. One of the first things Azeb does for new patients is show them her collection of before-and-after photographs. She points out one on the wall, of a shrunken little girl who looks like a Belsen victim. 'This one was fifteen. She had hardly any muscle left on her legs; bad contractures of the knee and hip. She couldn't even stand up when she arrived. We tried with a walking frame and gradually the muscles came back. She's had her fistula operation now and she's cured.'

Azeb points to a photograph of a woman standing up holding onto the wall. One knee is bent so that her toes barely touch the ground. 'This lady was 43 years old. There was no response to physio at first, so we used a plaster of Paris cast to extend the Achilles tendon. She was here for more than six months. She went home cured and walking properly.'

The girls prepare for sitting exercises. As they leave the bars they stagger and hold onto one another. One who has a walking frame has her foot dangling well clear of the ground. 'Most of them are depressed when they come here,' says Azeb. 'Then they see that there are others the same, and they feel a bit better.'

She takes me over to a woman sitting in a chair. 'She has a bad contracture of the knee. We tried for a few months with physio but we couldn't make it work, so we took her to the Black Lion [Hospital, in Addis Ababa] to see an orthopaedic surgeon. He said she has to have a tendon release. We'll keep her here a bit longer, then have it done. All of this has to happen before we can cure the fistula, so she's going to be here a long time.'

Every morning I've noticed one particular young woman shuffling past with the help of a walking stick. She always stands alone outside the physiotherapy department, holding onto a post doing leg exercises. Azeb introduces us. Her name is Lingersh. She's from Gojjam province and thinks she's about twenty. Her story is like a dozen others I've heard by now: a long labour, a stillbirth, incontinence both of urine and faeces. But there's a twist to this one which fills me with outrage. After three days of labour she was taken to a hospital at which the dead baby was delivered, but there was no explanation of why she was leaking. Instead they instructed her to come back in three months' time. Lingersh thought the fistula was due to something they'd done, so why should she go back?

At first she didn't even realise she had a fistula. Her main worry was her leg, which was giving her a lot of pain. When she discovered that she was leaking both urine and faeces, she was depressed and crying all the time. 'There's no way to express it,' she tells me.

Then her husband left her, so she just stayed in her parents' home, lying down without moving. After four months her brother took her to a local clinic near her village and there she heard about the new fistula hospital at Bahar Dar. Her brother and a friend carried her there and someone from the hospital drove her in the hospital car to Addis.

As Azeb translates for me she is unconsciously caressing Lingersh: adjusting her gown, rubbing her back, giving her a little hug now and then. Lingersh has had an operation to divert the bowel to a colostomy bag. When she can walk they'll do the fistula operation, then reverse the diversion. At first she was in a wheelchair, then had a walking frame and now she's nearly independent. Azeb is sure she'll walk normally again.

Simenesh is another member of that sad morning parade. She's nineteen and comes from the far west. She was in labour for five days. When I hear this I note it down without quite realising its significance, I've recorded so many histories by now. Then it strikes me – five days of labour! It's impossible to understand what an ordeal that must have been.

Simenesh is a big girl, not as fine-featured as most Ethiopians. She looks me in the eye when she speaks and smiles a lot – a broad, winsome smile. She spent two years lying on her side hoping that she'd get better. Some missionaries heard about her plight and brought her to the hospital on a stretcher. Azeb remembers that she was so ill with oedema and internal organ problems that they put her in intensive care at the Black Lion. The first day they tried to get her to sit up in bed she cried out in a panic because she was afraid of falling out. She'd never been in a bed before. When they brought her to the physiotherapy department in a wheelchair and she saw the photographs and met some other girls, she said, 'Now I have hope.'

Simenesh is a tough case. She's been here five months. She's had a temporary colostomy too, and it will probably be another five months before she's well enough to have her double fistula repaired.

I ask Simenesh and Lingersh if they would like to remarry when they are cured. They both reply with an emphatic 'No'. But the harsh truth for Ethiopian women is that they need to marry, for no other life is available to them. Azeb understands their feelings, though. 'Most of them don't want to remarry because the experience has been so bad. They are downhearted, they've lost their husband, their baby, everything. And also they have a fear whether they will be successfully cured, as most of them are waiting for surgery because they are so weak. When they are cured you see very different faces. You wonder if they are the same person.'

Reg used to tell patients when they were being discharged, 'You'll find another husband and have children. When you feel the baby walking around inside you, start walking to the hospital.'

Usually they take that advice. Sometimes former patients come back to show off their babies. When they do, Azeb makes sure that her girls see them. 'I remember one girl who had very bad contractures of the hip and knee. She was emaciated and weak when she came. She'd been lying still for eight months. After almost one year she was able to walk by herself. She had an operation and went home dry.

'This is her.' She shows me a photograph of a girl who looks like a skeleton. She has an old woman's wrinkled face but is only eighteen. 'She looks that way because of malnutrition,' says Azeb. 'She came back a little while ago with a beautiful one-year-old baby girl.'

Azeb believes there's no other place like this in the world to work. 'I'm very happy doing what I'm doing. We're here for one reason and that's helping women. It really gives me a good feeling.'

One of her most celebrated successes was a girl named Minsera, whom I'd met when I was last here. A good way to appreciate the miraculous change in her life is to read an abbreviated version of what Catherine wrote then.

Minsera is eighteen, but she is so slight that she looks like a child. One Sunday in 1998 I came back from church and found her lying on the couch in outpatients with a man standing beside her. She was frightened and in agony. Her left hip was completely dislocated and this leg was lying across the other one. It was impossible to examine her as I could not move her legs without her screaming with pain.

Minsera was from a village outside Harar. She had been in bed for five months and had bed sores right down to the bone on her back. The kind man who brought her told us she had an aunt and some relatives who fed her, but they didn't know what to do. He must have been a relative, I think. When he saw her he felt such pity for her that he decided to take her to Addis Ababa.

It is an all-day journey on the train from Harar and he carried her in his arms all the way. I don't know how he did it. He told us how, during her long labour, Minsera had been heaving on a rope attached to the roof of the hut to try and get purchase to push the baby out. The rope broke and she fell down, dislocating her hip. We were surprised that such a simple fall could do so much damage and were to discover the reason later.

Minsera was in a pitiful state – emaciated and dehydrated, her clothes soaked in urine and soiled with bowel contents. The smell in outpatients was overpowering. To lift her caused acute pain, so we gave her a very small injection of morphia and, when she was ready, cut away her ragged clothes and put her into a hot bath.

To see her lying in a clean bed in her blue nightgown, with a bed cradle to keep the heavy blankets off her injured leg brought tears to my eyes. Our nursing aides took her to their hearts and gave her loving care in the following weeks. She was very anaemic and needed blood transfusions to correct this. So thin was she that I could easily place her upper arm in the circle made by my thumb and index finger, with space to spare.

It was many weeks before we sought advice from the orthopaedic department at the leprosy hospital on how to treat her dislocated hip. They attempted to pull the head of the femur back into its socket by traction, putting a pin through the lower end of her femur to which weights were attached. But everything failed because her bone was diseased. Very soon an abscess formed and pus drained out. We cultured the discharge in our laboratory and grew the tuberculosis bacillus. So now we knew why her bones had been so fragile.

Later she developed ascites, an accumulation of fluid in the abdominal cavity, and from this we also grew the tuberculosis bacillus, thus confirming that Minsera had disseminated TB. Fortunately her lungs remained clear, and chest X-rays were normal.

Our physician, Dr Amha, prescribed five different anti-TB drugs which, after eight months, completely cured the disease. As time went by her condition improved dramatically. Her appetite returned, she gained weight, her hair, which was thin and sparse like a soft down when she arrived, became thick and shiny. Her eyes sparkled and lit up her pretty little face as she now greeted everyone with a smile. We were able to do a colostomy once the ascites disappeared, and soon she learned to manage this and keep herself clean.

As soon as Minsera was strong enough, we started physiotherapy. I shall never forget the first day she got out of bed. We were all nervous about her taking this step, wondering what would happen to her hip. We were encouraged by a physiotherapist, Jenny Bassford, who happened to be with us on one of her annual visits from England to help in the newly established department.

It was marvellous to see Minsera standing by her bed supported by two of her devoted nursing aides. It was not long before she was taking a few steps with a walking frame for support, then with just two sticks.

Minsera's left hip has been completely destroyed, but it has become stable and is now ankylosed, which of course greatly restricts mobility. We have had her left shoe built up so that both her legs are the same length, and she now has no limp. Now as I write, two years after she arrived, she has just one stick and she does not always use even that.

Sadly, none of the vaginal operations have been possible yet. Because of her stiff hip joint we are not able to turn her left leg outwards. Access to the injuries is at present impossible. However, she is persevering with the physiotherapy and making tremendous progress. We are hopeful that soon there will be enough movement in that hip to enable us to repair her huge rectal defect and close the colostomy. Later she will need an ileal conduit, as her whole bladder has been destroyed. There is no tissue to repair.

The last chapter of Minsera's story has not yet been written, but even so far the tale is remarkable. When I first saw her lying on that outpatients' couch I imagined we would just be trying to relieve her suffering for a few days until her death. Her recovery to this stage is almost totally due to the devoted nursing care given by our staff. Doctors walk around giving orders and prescribing drugs, but the daily task of looking after an emaciated, incontinent girl with bed sores and an excruciatingly painful hip has demanded nursing skills and compassion of the highest order.

Now the last chapter *can* be written. Minsera is a nurse aide herself. One evening when I know she is on night duty, I go looking for her in the main ward. The sister in charge tells me she is in another ward a short walk away. She asks a nursing sister who speaks English to take me to Minsera.

We are about 50 metres away walking along the covered pathway to the ward when the sister starts shouting, 'Minsera, Minsera!' followed by a torrent of Amharic.

There is an answering shout and they keep up a running conversation at the top of their voices as we approach. The last time I'd seen Minsera she was a frail little girl sitting on the edge of a bed with her stick legs dangling. She looked feeble and listless. Now I am stunned to see a beautiful, vibrant young woman walking towards us. She has not yet changed into her uniform, and is wearing a long pale blue dress which hides her built-up shoe, a pretty cotton jumper in blue and white, and a royal blue headscarf with a white pattern. She has big silver earrings. It's all beautifully coordinated. Minsera's face lights up with a vivacious smile.

I explain that I was here seven years ago when she was very sick and that I am writing a book. I ask her if she remembers what she was like then – tentatively, because I don't want to make her unhappy. She smiles sweetly. 'I was very sick.'

'How do you feel now?'

'I am very happy.' Well, you can see that. I don't really want to interrogate her. It's enough just to see her. Everything that needs to be said is there in front of me, in her glowing good health and her bright personality.

Minsera's village was near Harar, where they're building another fistula hospital. When it opens she'll go there to work. I ask if I can take a photograph and she poses cheekily in front of some patients. The flash goes off and they all gather round to exclaim over the picture. I leave feeling foolishly happy.

CHAPTER 5

Dinner this evening is at Catherine's house down the hill from the hospital complex. To get there you have to negotiate a pathway of raised concrete stepping stones, then a steep descent down unevenly spaced steps. It's an obstacle course for anyone, let alone a woman of Catherine's age, yet she sees no reason to have the access upgraded.

The whitewashed walls of the house are made of sticks plastered with mud mixed with wheat stalks. Over the years they've sagged a bit here and there and the doors are always a little hard to close. Inside, entertaining happens in a big main room which Catherine calls the drawing room. It's furnished with a couch and several comfortable chairs. In one corner there's a grand piano. On the closed lid is a framed black-and-white photograph of Reg Hamlin, taken, I would guess, when he was in his late forties. There are a few watercolours of Australian and Ethiopian land-scapes on the walls.

The meal has been prepared by Catherine's housekeeper, Yeshi. Yeshi's been with her since she was a teenage girl. She's in her sixties now. She's never hinted at retiring, but this year has been given an assistant, Birru's daughter, Zawdiresh. Birru has been working for Catherine for more than four decades, he's very much a part of her Ethiopian family. Zawdiresh will need to learn how to cook plain, old-fashioned English fare for Catherine.

Ruth is there, of course; and Dr Andrew Browning, an Australian who runs the hospital at Bahar Dar, is down for a visit. The conversation turns to Australia, where, it turns out, Ruth's brother is living. She's visited him at home but she says she could never live there because she can't speak the language. This inspires Catherine to tell a joke.

After the fall of Singapore in the Second World War, a wounded British serviceman comes to Darwin for treatment. He says to the nurse, 'I suppose I've come here to die.'

'No,' she replies. 'You came here yesterdai.'

It's so silly that it gets a good laugh. It works all the better due to Catherine's rather proper accent.

Andrew tells a story about a patient who came recently to Bahar Dar from out in the bush. Seeing her reflection in a mirror she said, 'That lady looks just like my sister.'

She then asked the image, 'How are you?'

Receiving no reply she tried again. When there was still no response she became indignant. 'Why isn't she speaking to me? Oh, this woman is so rude.'

Andrew tells another one about an old lady who came to the hospital after having a fistula for decades. As they wheeled her into the theatre she said, 'I don't care what happens to me now. I can die happy. I've slept in a bed and I've seen an electric light.'

He has yet another, concerning a woman from the Gumuz tribe over in the western part of the country near Sudan. The Gumuz are very dark people, much darker than the Amharas, who are the predominant group around Bahar Dar. She was in outpatients when she spied a black doll they use for teaching placed on top of a cupboard. 'Why are you ignoring this baby?' she demanded indignantly. 'Is it just because it's black?'

These days Catherine is preoccupied with managing the rapid expansion that's going on. She and Reg did 300 operations in their first year. This year the number will reach 3000. There's a proposal afoot to build an executive wing with offices for Catherine; the Medical Director, Dr Mulu Muleta; and the CEO, Mark Bennett; plus a conference room. Catherine's appalled at the idea. 'It's ridiculous to think that I need my own office. I've made do with a desk in the drawing room for thirty years.'

That's true, although there has been one change since I was here last – the addition of a laptop computer. She's learnt how to use e-mail – sort of. She complains that sometimes things seem to disappear, then calls Ruth to come and help her get them back again. She has not yet mastered the internet. She still writes several letters a week in longhand and bemoans the loss of this traditional way of communicating.

The trustees are in the process of buying a new block of land just down the hill from the hospital. Someone has suggested that they put in a road. Catherine is outraged about that, too. 'Can you imagine? A ghastly great road. Think what it will cost. Over my dead body.'

There is a moment of silence – just a fraction of a second more than would be natural – before the conversation starts up again. Her words raise a spectre that everyone at the hospital is thinking about but no one wants to mention.

Two weeks before Christmas 2006 Catherine came down with what seemed to be a heavy cold. She decided to stay in bed at home to try to shake it off. At first no one at the hospital was too worried about her, but on about the third day her condition began to worsen. The heavy cold had turned into pneumonia.

The doctors at the hospital were looking after her, advised by the very competent physician, Dr Amha, who has a contract with the hospital. Catherine has an insurance policy that allows for medical evacuation in the case of critical illness. Mark Bennett asked the doctors if they thought evacuation would be necessary. They told him that at this stage they didn't think so. They felt that they were managing adequately with antibiotics.

Next day her condition was much worse. She had developed septicaemia, or blood poisoning, and was running a high fever. She was delirious and didn't know where she was. When Dr Haile, with whom she'd worked for eight years, went to see her she didn't recognise him. He came out of her bedroom and burst into tears.

It was clearly time for more drastic intervention. Catherine was taken to the Black Lion Hospital and placed in intensive care. Mark, meanwhile, contacted the health insurance company in the UK to enquire about a medical evacuation. They advised him that Catherine's policy called for evacuation to her home country or 'the nearest point of good medical care'. Australia was too far to go in her present serious condition, so Mark suggested that they take her to the UK. She could go to Hammersmith Hospital in London, where they know her well from previous stays. Perhaps more importantly, her son, Richard, lived in London. No one knew what the coming days might bring. If the worst happened, this might be the last chance she'd have to see him.

The insurance company told Mark that the UK was not an option. The nearest point of good medical care was Johannesburg in South Africa. This created a dilemma for Mark. Even if the medical care was first class, he wasn't happy about sending her off at her age to a foreign country where she didn't know anyone and there'd be no one from the Fistula Hospital to follow her up. They'd told him that the plane was only big enough to carry the doctor and nurses, so someone, probably Ruth, would have to follow on a commercial flight. That might take a couple of days. The only other option was for the hospital to pay the £80,000 cost of the evacuation to London.

What followed was the most stressful 24 hours in Mark Bennett's life. He had been at the hospital for only eighteen months, and he was being called upon to make possibly a life-or-death decision about its beloved founder, Dr Hamlin. A key part of his job was to ensure that donated funds were scrupulously managed. 'I felt that it was an enormous amount of money that people had given for the treatment of patients and before we used it for the treatment of one of our staff, even if it was our founder, we ought to just make sure we were spending it in the right way.'

In his previous life Mark had been an executive at Arnott's Biscuits in Sydney. His time in the corporate world had taught him that no matter what the outcome, questions would be asked later. This wasn't a decision that he could make alone. He asked the chairman of the hospital trust, a retired banker, Ato Tekalign Gedamu, to come and sit with him while he made a round of telephone calls to trustees in the UK, America and Australia. It was the middle of the night for some of them. The answers were unanimous – spend the money.

Mark gave the go-ahead. In the meantime Catherine was not responding to any of the antibiotics that were available at the Black Lion. Her prognosis was looking grim. Fourteen hours after Mark had given the green light a plane which was virtually a flying intensive care ward landed at Addis Ababa. On board were a doctor and a nurse, both women. They were Swiss – very Germanic Swiss, is how Ruth remembers them.

'They're not like our wonderful Ethiopian staff, are they?' Catherine whispered as they carried her on board. They were certainly very efficient, Ruth recalls, but the bedside manner left a bit to be desired.

When they took off, Ruth was also a passenger. Seeing as they were paying, Mark had insisted that she be included.

For the staff left behind at the hospital it was an anxious night.

Many of them were wondering if they would ever see Catherine again. At three o'clock in the morning Mark received a call from the doctor on the plane in Libya. They had stopped at Benghazi to refuel and were trying to decide where to go next. There was heavy fog in London and commercial flights were being diverted. The Swiss were advocating Zurich, quite possibly because they wanted to get home for Christmas. There was no question about the standard of care there but Ruth was not happy about subjecting Catherine to more Germanic-style 'compassion'. Mark had been impressed by the American hospital in Paris when he'd taken his daughter there about a year earlier. After a round of phone calls between Mark and the evacuation team, that was where they decided to go.

The plane landed in mid-morning and just a few hours later in Addis they got the news that everyone had been praying for. Catherine was responding well to very powerful antibiotics. Her condition had stabilised and things were looking a lot better.

Mark still wanted to get her to London, but first he had another long tussle with the insurance company about who would pay for it. Initially they declined to meet the cost, but after a lot of persuasion they agreed that it was up to them to get her there.

An ambulance came across the Channel to pick them up. With Catherine, Ruth and a doctor on board, they set off for Calais. You could almost describe the trip that followed as a comedy, if the situation hadn't been so serious. The two drivers were, in Ruth's words, 'two rather blobby young men who were a disaster waiting to happen'. First they lost their way trying to find the main road to Calais. Then the heating in the patient's section of the ambulance failed. The glass dividing the drivers from the back was removed and their heating was turned up to full. They wrapped Catherine in aluminium foil and blankets.

Once they found the main road there seemed to be nothing else that could go wrong – until they ran out of fuel, just managing to coast to an SOS call box. Fortunately Ruth speaks French, so she was able to explain their predicament to the emergency team. They negotiated the Channel Tunnel without incident, then, about an hour from London, there was another delay when the oxygen ran out and had to be replaced with a spare cylinder. Finally, when they were unloading Catherine at Hammersmith Hospital the head section of the stretcher suddenly dropped and she suffered a minor whiplash injury.

For the first few days in Hammersmith she was so weak that she could not walk. Ruth remained constantly by her side. As a trained nurse she was well able to help Catherine with such things as sit-down showers, washing her hair, and so on. They prayed together and when the patient was up to it, they had some good laughs over the ambulance journey from hell.

Ten days after being admitted, Catherine was well enough to be discharged. She went to stay with Richard at his London home. With her son, daughter-in-law and four grandchildren to look after her, she slowly regained her strength. At the end of January she was well enough to return home.

Catherine and I are sitting on the couch in her drawing room drinking Yeshi's strong coffee, nibbling biscuits which someone has brought from England. 'Did you think you were going to die?' I ask.

'I didn't think I was going to die. They all thought I was going to die, but I thought I'd get better. When I came back there was a terrific party. I said, "Now don't give me a party until the afternoon." Ruth and Edjigayehu [the Matron] organised it, a huge do in the chapel here. I was very touched by that.'

'They do love you, don't they?' I venture.

'They do. They do love me and I love them too. It's mutual.'

The affection for Catherine Hamlin spreads wider than among her staff. The bill from the Black Lion Hospital for her time in intensive care came to 4 birr – about 50 Australian cents.

CHAPTER 6

When Catherine and Reg first came to Ethiopia it was like a feudal kingdom in the Middle Ages. The country was ruled by the emperor, Haile Selassie. Said to be descended from King Solomon, his full title was: Conquering Lion of the Tribe of Judah, King of Kings of Ethiopia and Elect of God. The emperor was surrounded by the sort of opulence one would expect of an absolute monarch. There was a privileged aristocracy who lived in ostentatious splendour. By contrast, the majority of people were subsistence farmers, many of whom existed on the edge of starvation.

The women Catherine and Reg cared for at the Princess Tsehai Hospital were invariably penniless. But the Hamlins were also required to attend the births of wealthy private patients, and occasionally women from the palace. These patients would have private rooms set aside for them, and would arrive with carpets, furniture and servants to attend to their needs. These days Catherine occasionally meets socially people whom she delivered into the world back then.

In Addis Ababa the Hamlins were part of a small expatriate community. They went to embassy dinners, gymkhanas, and lunches, attended performances by the Amateur Dramatic Society and sometimes the christenings of babies they had delivered. Catherine owned horses, and she and Richard often rode out into the countryside which came right to their doorstep. Catherine was friends with several of the princesses. The emperor visited the hospital occasionally, and now and then they were invited to the palace – once for Reg to receive a humanitarian award for his services to the Ethiopian people.

Haile Selassie had a fondness for lions, one or two of which used to roam at will in the palace gardens. He was also rumoured to keep one chained up outside his reception rooms, something which Catherine found hard to believe until she arranged an audience with His Majesty for two benefactors from Australia. Sure enough, there was a lion in the hallway. It sat quite passively while the visitors gave it a pat.

In 1960, while the emperor was out of the country visiting Brazil, the head of the imperial bodyguard staged a revolt. Catherine was in the labour ward delivering a baby when there was the sound of gunfire and a volley of bullets flew past the window. The nurse assisting her fled, leaving Catherine alone in the midst of a forceps delivery. Fortunately for patient and baby, she returned in time to help complete the procedure.

Reg had gone to collect Richard from school. As they drove through the centre of town they were fired upon. They made a quick detour into the Ministry of Commerce building, where they spent the next several hours hiding under a table.

During a lull in the fighting they made a dash for home and arrived unscathed. Their house in the grounds of the government hospital was in a no-man's-land between forces loyal to the emperor, and the rebels. The family huddled in the hall, which seemed the safest place, while the fighting raged, occasionally flinching when bullets lodged in the walls of the house.

Catherine and Reg spent four days practically without sleep, as they helped the general surgeons attend to dozens of people who had been wounded in the fighting. In the end the loyalists got the upper hand. The emperor returned home in triumph and the three leaders of the revolt were publicly hanged, two in the main square and one outside the hospital gates. For the next few days, as Richard went to and from school, he had to pass the body turning slowly in the breeze.

By 1974 they had bought the land for the Fistula Hospital and raised enough money to build the first rudimentary structures. There was a building containing the ward with 40 beds, an operating theatre, changing rooms, storerooms and an office where the doctors could write up their notes. Another small building housed the kitchen and laundry and some rooms for live-in staff.

It was an unstable time politically. Ethiopia was in the grip of a devastating famine, in which hundreds of thousands of people had starved to death. Students had begun openly to protest against the monarchy. Things came to a head when a group of young army officers, calling themselves the Armed Forces Co-ordinating Committee, later known as the *Dergue*, arrested politicians, the emperor's courtiers and advisers, members of the imperial family and many nobles and prominent landowners.

Haile Selassie's demise was heralded on television screens on the night of Ethiopian New Year. The whole nation was invited to watch a television documentary in which the producers cleverly juxtaposed images of lavish banquets alongside shots of peasants starving in the famine. One sequence showed the extravagant wedding of a nobleman's daughter, complete with an imported wedding cake said to have cost $3000. Shots of the emperor feeding his dogs were interposed with pictures of dying children.

The day following the emperor's humiliation on television, soldiers went to the palace to inform him of his dethronement. Reg and Catherine, staunch monarchists both, took Haile Selassie's downfall hard. They did not believe the charges of corruption against him. There was little they could do except keep their heads down and hope that the new regime would be as kindly disposed to them as the old.

A year after his arrest, Haile Selassie was murdered by his captors. The *Dergue*'s aim was to turn Ethiopia into a communist state along the lines of Stalinist Russia. The wealthy were stripped of their homes and land, and ordinary middle-class people had their businesses confiscated and handed over to the state. Churches were closed and many missionaries thrown out of the country. Those who remained were often persecuted, and in some cases murdered.

A network of spies informed on anyone who spoke out against the *Dergue*. It became common to hear gunshots in the night and to see bodies in the street, left lying there as a lesson to others who might be contemplating rebellion. Once Catherine was on her way to pick up some medical supplies when she came across a pile of bodies stripped naked and tossed in a pile onto a vacant block of land. They were victims of so-called 'revolutionary justice'. She was so shocked that she could not go on. She stopped to regain her composure, then turned around and went home.

Reg and Catherine watched these developments with alarm, never knowing if the hospital was about to be taken over, or if they themselves would be harmed. Catherine thinks the reason they were allowed to keep going without interference during the seventeen years of communist rule was that they were treating the poor for free. They did not cost the government anything and were not making any profit for themselves.

Some of the princesses and their relatives were imprisoned, first of all in a vermin-infested cell, then in a special political prison, where eleven women were confined to one room. Bravely, Catherine never made any secret of her friendship with the royal family. Every Sunday after church she used to take them presents of cake and biscuits, or marmalade she had made. She was also able to pass on books and food that friends in England had sent. Although she was not allowed to see the prisoners face to face, they were able to secrete notes when they returned the food utensils. Then Catherine would relay their needs to supporters in the outside world.

As the years of terrorism and oppression dragged on, rebel groups based in Tigray province began harassing the Ethiopian army. By the late 1980s the country was embroiled in full-scale civil war, with terrible casualties on both sides.

By early 1991 the rebel forces, led by the man who is now prime minister, Meles Zenawi, were pushing down from the north, driving the Ethiopian army before them. On 28 May the city was blacked out and Catherine and Reg could hear gunfire close to the hospital. Realising that his time was up, Major Mengistu, military leader of the *Dergue*, fled in a light plane to seek sanctuary with his pal Robert Mugabe in Zimbabwe.

On the day the rebels took Addis Ababa, Catherine was knitting on a couch in her house when the telephone rang. She got up to answer it. It was a friend, Pippa Sandford, asking her if she was coming to the British Embassy as had been advised.

Catherine told Pippa that she would stay where she was, as she didn't want to leave the patients.

Just at that moment a bullet came through the ceiling and lodged in the cushion where Catherine had been sitting. Pippa, still on the other end of the line, heard the noise and Catherine's exclamation of alarm: 'Oh, Pippa, you may have just saved my life.'

Catherine and Reg survived the communist regime by being scrupulously non-political. The same approach has worked with the current government. The present system could hardly be described as a democracy. The weeks leading up to the 2005 elections were marked by violence and intimidation against opposition candidates. Observers from the European Union reported more than 300 cases of opposition activists being beaten, threats and intimidation against supporters of opposition parties, and isolated cases of murder. The EU noted that just before the elections the penal code had been altered so that the news media was restricted in their reporting, and organisations wanting to act as domestic electoral observers were banned. The week before election day hundreds of opposition supporters were arrested or went missing and several young political activists from the opposition were killed during violent clashes with government supporters.

The day after the election the government declared a state of emergency in the capital and imposed a month-long ban on demonstrations. When votes were counted, opposition candidates had won every seat in Addis Ababa, and won constituencies over large areas of the country. Yet the government was returned to power. The two main opposition parties charged that the process was fraudulent and demanded that a new poll be held.

In Addis, members of the opposition refused to take their seats in the parliament, charging that the democratic process would not be observed. They asked their supporters to stage a day of protest by staying away from work and burning rubber tyres at certain points in the city. The federal police were mobilised to stop them and there were a number of violent clashes.

Ruth was showing two Japanese women through the hospital that day. They had a clear view across the river to a street where students were burning tyres and throwing stones at police. Suddenly they saw them open fire and shoot two protesters dead. Not surprisingly, the visitors were very upset.

In October 2006 an independent investigation by an Ethiopian judge, Wolde-Michael Meshesha, found that 193 protesters, including 40 teenagers, had been killed. Police records showed that 20,000 people were arrested during the protests. More than 100 opposition leaders, journalists and aid workers were imprisoned and charged with treason and attempted genocide. The judge has since fled Ethiopia.

It's a great tribute to the Hamlins that they have been able to deal successfully with a succession of rulers, from the emperor, Haile Selassie, through the time of the murderous and unpredictable *Dergue*, to the present volatile regime. Stories of missions and non-government organisations (NGOs) having difficulties are legion, yet for half a century Catherine has sailed serenely through the political storms, not only surviving but thriving. The current government, it must be said, has been generous to a fault. They donated the land on which Desta Mender ('Joy Village' in Amharic) was recently built. Desta Mender is a village about 10 kilometres from the hospital housing women with chronic long-term injuries which prevent them from returning home. Catherine has always had good access to the Minister for Health if she needs it, and he has proven to be a sympathetic supporter.

Living in Ethiopia has had a personal cost. Richard had an idyllic childhood, with freedom and space, friends from a dozen different nationalities to play with, and his mother and father always there. Yet it was a testing one, too. Not many western children have dodged bullets and seen bodies hanging from the gallows as they made their way to school, or shaken hands with emperors.

When Richard reached high school age, his parents debated whether to send him to day school in Ethiopia; in Australia, where he could have lived with one of Catherine's siblings; or to boarding school in England. Travel to and from Australia was difficult and expensive, so they decided on England. At the age of fourteen Richard exchanged the carefree life he had known for the harsh discipline, the loneliness and schoolboy cruelties of an English boarding school. In his words, 'I went straight from Ethiopia and sunshine to a winter and a load of boys who didn't care a fig about me.'

He tried to be brave about it. In an early letter home he wrote:

> I am afraid I was a rather weak-willed Christian for the first few days and did not have the guts to get down on my knees at night and pray, but I remembered all you told me and what God thinks of me and have prayed on my knees every night for the last week.

A more worldly child might have known that it would not pay to be so defiantly different. With the wisdom of adulthood, Richard says, 'It makes me wince when I think of it. Not because I'm ashamed of saying my prayers, but it was done with such "I'm going to show them" conviction. I'm sure it did impress some people secretly, but there are ways and ways of doing things. It became part of my identity.'

Richard's three years at boarding school were miserable. Touchy, sensitive, lonely, he was a natural target for bullies. He reacted by fairly regularly picking fights to defend himself.

It was Reg's fondest desire that his son would study medicine and one day take over running the hospital. Richard dutifully enrolled in the medical school attached to St Bartholomew's Hospital in London but very soon began to wonder if medicine was what he really wanted to do. For the sake of his father he persevered, but as the course wore on he found himself filled with dread at the mere thought of having to face patients. To try to gain some semblance of control over his life he embarked upon a regime of rigorous physical training. He soon began to suffer from anorexia due to his internal conflict. Once, he fainted from hunger in an operating theatre. In faraway Ethiopia his parents did not realise that he was going through a debilitating emotional crisis.

Reg and Catherine told Richard to come home for a while, and the three of them spent long hours discussing his future. He told his father that he wanted to give up medicine and do a science course. But Reg thought that, having come so far, it would be unwise to drop out now and urged him to complete his degree.

Should they have listened more closely to their son? This is easy to say but it must be remembered that at the same time Richard was considering his future Reg and Catherine were consumed with all the arrangements for opening the new hospital and Major Mengistu was embarking on his murderous reign of terror. They gave Richard the advice they considered right at the time. He returned to London and, as he knew he would, failed his exams.

He took a year off, doing labouring work in London, then returned to study for his finals once more. As the months went by, again he wrestled with conflicting emotions, his heart telling him that he disliked medicine, but loyalty to his father keeping him going with it. At the eleventh hour he decided that he could pretend no more and wrote home saying that he was quitting medicine for good. Reg was devastated at the news; his cherished ambition was shattered. He wrote urging Richard to reconsider, but there was no going back.

When I was researching *The Hospital by the River* in 2000 I had heard hints of this story from some of Catherine's friends in Australia. In Addis Ababa I asked Catherine about it. At first she did not want to talk about it at all, it was just too painful. Then, a few days later, after having thought some more, she changed her mind. She had come to the view that if we were to write an honest account of her life, the story of Richard's emotional crisis could not be left out. She had kept the letters he wrote home at that time and now, bravely, she offered to read some extracts to me. They were full of pain and longing, Richard's confusion and guilt laid bare. In one, he told his parents how in the preceding month he had twice been overcome by excruciating grief. He thought that these episodes were not hysterical or emotional, but arose out of a deep longing to see his father again.

After Richard abandoned medicine he got a job in the fledgling IT industry. He married Diana Cliff, a sweet and supportive young woman who was a nurse at St Bartholomew's Hospital. They went on to have four children. Father and son wrote occasional letters but did not see each other for the next seven years. Then, at Christmas 1984 Richard, Diana and their first two children went to Ethiopia for a visit. Richard vividly remembers seeing his father again. 'It was as though nothing had happened. I saw Dad and he was waving from the airport viewing place. We embraced and kissed and it all came back together. We'd written a bit during the seven years. I went back more regularly after that, but I did detect frustration in Dad, whether it was about me doing medicine or about my IT career which was just getting going, but he was very keen for me to succeed. That was part of his makeup. We always got on well despite that. There were no harsh words. The rift had been bad for both of us.'

CHAPTER 7

One morning, two days after Catherine has operated on Amina, I go to the main ward to see how she's getting on. She's lying in bed with the blanket pulled up to her chin, looking pretty sorry for herself. Because of the repair to her rectum she hasn't been allowed to eat for two days, and she's hungry. She brightens up a bit when she's told that she'll be able to start on a light diet tomorrow and then gradually work up to the standard hospital menu.

I call on Zemebech, Dr Abiy's patient. She's chatting with another girl from Wollo province. She feels good, she says, and the nurse tells me that the bed is dry, which is a good sign. Zemebech says she was very frightened going into the theatre, but now that the surgery has been done she's much happier.

Abiy tells me that hers was the most difficult operation he's ever done but he feels cautiously confident that she will be cured. The critical time will be on about the fourteenth post-operative day, when they remove the catheter draining her bladder.

Abiy's still mulling over Catherine's offer to become a fistula surgeon. No doubt one of the things he's weighing up is the difference in the salary he'll earn if he forsakes private practice for a less lucrative career working for poor rural women. If he does decide to be a fistula surgeon it will be for all the right reasons.

Another of the patients who had surgery that day, Halema, from Somalia, is talking to a Somali man. He was visiting someone else and heard there was another Somali patient, so he came over for a chat. As he speaks Amharic this is a good opportunity to find out more of Halema's story.

She lives in a part of Somalia that is wracked by war. When she heard that there was a hospital in Ethiopia which could repair her fistula, she and her sister walked for two days from her village to the border. Then they waited until a group of Somalis was crossing and asked if they could go with them. On the other side they found someone who could speak their language and asked for directions to Addis Ababa. They spent another five days on the road getting here. There's a sizeable Somali community in Addis and they all look after one another. Her sister will be staying with them until Halema is ready to go home.

Halema is feeling well and the bed is dry. When I ask her what she'll do when she leaves here, she says she doesn't want to marry. 'I just want to live a healthy life.' Then, for some reason, she and her visitor crack up with laughter. Here is a woman whose husband has died, she's lost her only baby and is unlikely ever to have another chance at motherhood; she's had a fistula, is in hospital in a country where no one speaks her language, and she can laugh. Her spirit is amazing.

Dr Habte's patient, Letelibanes, is lying in bed in the post-operative ward. Lete has an Ethiopian cross tattooed on her forehead and four rows of tattoos around her neck and across her chest. The blanket is pulled up to her chin, and her fingers are peeping out from under it. There are a few flecks of red polish left on her nails. Her fingers wiggle and wave and she raises her eyes – big, expressive eyes – heavenwards to emphasise her points.

With Habte translating, she tells me her story. She says that some time after the birth of her son she felt a stone inside her. It was so painful that her parents thought she was going to die. After about a year she passed it and then felt much better.

Dr Habte thinks this was probably a bladder stone. He once photographed one that was 20 centimetres across, which they had to crush to get out. Habte goes into a long, technical description of Lete's operation. The bottom line is that the fistula has been closed, but there was quite a bit of scarring, which is not good. That, plus her short urethra and small bladder, makes him suspect that she might have some stress incontinence. At the moment there's a catheter draining her bladder. If she's still dry after fourteen days the big test will come when they remove the catheter.

When Lete got the fistula her husband deserted her and her son. She was afraid, left alone in his village without any relatives, so she made the two-hour walk back to her parents' home, which is where she's been living. Lete says she lived with the fistula for three years and then her mother took her to the new fistula centre at Mekele. It was a six-hour walk to the road and then three days in a series of buses. At Mekele they told her that her injury was too severe to be treated there. They recommended that she go to Addis Ababa, but she was afraid to go by herself, so she waited at Mekele until there was another patient. The people at the hospital gave them the bus fare and the two of them went to Addis together.

Up until now she's seemed quite happy. When I ask her how the fistula affected her life, there's a change. Her chin trembles and her eyes glisten; I think she's about to burst into tears. 'No one came to see me,' she says. 'The neighbours looked at me as though I might have a disease. I spent all the time inside hiding.'

I ask Lete how she feels now. At first she thinks I'm asking about her medical condition. Then Habte explains. 'I am happy,' she says. 'I am thanking God.'

I go looking for Alganish, whom I'd met a few days ago when she arrived at outpatients. There are four wards at the Fistula Hospital, each in a separate building. She's in the Betel ward, down the hill between the kitchen and the laundry, where patients live while they're waiting for their operations. The rain hasn't yet begun so they're all outside enjoying the sun. Alganish is by herself, crouching on the ground with her shawl draped over her head, spilling down around her, arms thrust out straight, the upper parts resting on her knees, hands dangling. The crouching woman; a classic Ethiopian tableau. She smiles sweetly when she sees me. Although my translators have explained what I'm here for, I'm not at all sure she understands the concept of writing a book. I suspect she thinks I'm a doctor. She says she's still worried about her husband not looking after his stepchildren, but she's happy to be here with the hope of a cure. She's fasting, as her operation is scheduled for tomorrow.

My last visit is to Leteabazgi, who had arrived on the same day as Alganish. She still has a shy, introverted manner, and doesn't have much to say. Her operation hasn't been scheduled yet, so she's just waiting. She seems overwhelmed by everything that's happening to her. Understandably. Before her ill-fated pregnancy, life was simple and her future predictable. Now she doesn't know what's in store for her.

I feel I'm getting to know these women whom I've chosen randomly to track. And I can feel something happening that I'd rather hoped to avoid. I'm becoming involved.

There's always a lot of activity in the wards during daylight hours. Doctors are doing rounds, nurse aides are constantly mopping the floors, nursing sisters are attending to the needs of recuperating patients. One of the dearest and oldest workers, Letebirhan, whom I met on my last visit, is still here, circulating around in her wheelchair. Lete lives in the ward with all her worldly possessions beside her bed in a small chest of drawers. She arrived from Axum, in the north of the country, a few years after Reg and Catherine began working in Ethiopia. As we recounted in *The Hospital by the River*, her fistula was not caused by childbirth. Lete was betrothed as a young girl, and then it was discovered that she had an imperforate hymen. The *wogesha* was called. During the 'operation' he cut through her urethra and bladder, thus causing her to suffer from complete incontinence and a fistula. The hospital mended her injuries but the experience she had suffered was so traumatic that she decided she did not want to marry and stayed on to help. Some time later she was knocked down by a car and broke her back. She is paralysed from the waist down.

For many years Lete helped out in the operating theatre, then, when the physiotherapy department opened, was trained by a visiting English physiotherapist. She goes around the ward in her wheelchair chatting to patients, listening sympathetically to their troubles, counselling them, and helping them with exercises to relieve atrophied muscles and contractions of the joints.

At night the windows in the main ward are closed, the curtains are drawn and most of the activity ceases. One evening at about

8 pm I pop in to have a chat to the sister in charge, Sister Almaz. She's one of several people who have been working with Catherine since the old days at Princess Tsehai. Once people come to the Fistula Hospital they rarely want to work anywhere else.

There's something going on up near the entrance. A mobile screen has been placed around one of the beds and I can see several people clustered around the patient. Except that it's not a patient – they're laying out the body of Mama Mulu, an old beggar woman, probably in her late eighties, who has been coming to the hospital for her meals for fifteen years. A family who lives up the road gave Mama Mulu a place to sleep, and she'd arrive at the hospital every lunchtime for a plate of *injera* and *wat*, the same meal that the patients have. She'd take something home with her for her evening meal.

Five weeks ago the people who had taken her in had sent word that she was very sick. She had lived way longer than the average person in Ethiopia, despite her desperately hard existence, and her exhausted old body was finally giving up. She'd suffered a series of medical problems, the most recent of which had been a stroke two weeks previously, which had paralysed her right side. The hospital had given her a bed and made her last days as comfortable and painless as possible.

Next day Ruth finds some money and sends one of the drivers, Hamid, out to buy a box. Sister Almaz tracks down a priest and the hospital pays for the funeral. Some of the hospital staff who've known Mama Mulu go to pay their respects. Mama Mulu had no possessions and no living relatives that anyone knew of. But there are people to mourn her and bury her, so in the end she has as much as the richest person in the land.

CHAPTER 8

Catherine is excited because her brother, Jock Nicholson, and his wife, Louise, have come for a visit. Jock, the youngest of Catherine's five siblings, is a farmer in Limbri, near Tamworth, New South Wales. And he looks it. He has a ruddy complexion and favours tweed jackets and brogues. Even on holiday he wears a tie.

The day after they arrive, Jock, Louise, Catherine, Ruth and I go to church together. St Matthew's is Anglican. It was opened in 1955, four years before Reg and Catherine arrived in Ethiopia. Catherine has always worshipped there. As the hospital Toyota pulls up outside, a line of beggars stirs against the church wall. Catherine carries a collection of small change with her. She goes along the line depositing coins into each grimy hand.

The congregation is partly European and partly African. There are a lot of aid workers and embassy people; everyone seems to know everyone else. It's a conventional Anglican service, with old-fashioned, time-tested hymns – none of your modern happy-clappy stuff. After the service is over and we're having tea on the lawn, a steady stream of friends comes up to wish Catherine well.

We go off to lunch at one of Addis Ababa's smart restaurants, in an open-air terrace on the roof of a three-storey building. The patrons are a well-to-do crowd; a lot of them know Catherine and come up to talk.

The conversation turns to churches. Ruth tells an allegedly true story about a Scottish church service in which the plates go around and come back in the same state as when they had left. The minister holds them up, raises his eyes heavenward and says, 'Thank you, Lord, for the safe return of these plates.'

Jock tops this with a joke about an old lady with an ear trumpet going into a Scottish church. The minister, thinking it's a musical instrument, is reluctant to allow her in. She explains that it's an ear trumpet. 'Very well,' he says. 'You can come in, but one toot and ye're oot.'

Jock is a no-frills sort of bloke – straightforward, honest, and not at all worldly. He'd be eaten alive in the city, but at home on the farm, or here with Catherine, where the old values of decency and compassion still hold sway, he fits right in. Jock and Catherine's father was a wealthy man who made his fortune from manufacturing elevators. He and their mother were serious about their religion, and raised their children to have old-fashioned Christian values. Their father contributed to many charitable causes; their mother was so worried about the souls of the local children that she had a hall built in the grounds of the family home at Ryde so they'd have somewhere to attend Sunday school, which Catherine often taught. Louise is a trained nurse and has the same values as her husband. When Desta Mender, the village for incurable patients, was opened in 2003, Catherine thought that Jock and Louise would be the ideal people to run it.

About 8 per cent of the women who come to the Fistula Hospital are so badly injured that they can't be cured. Some have no bladder left at all, or they're so scarred that surgical repair is impossible. The solution is a urinary diversion. The most common is an 'ileal conduit': a section of the small intestine, the ileum, is removed; one end is closed and the ureters are inserted into the side. The other end is stitched to the abdominal wall with a 'stoma' to which a collection bag is attached. The bag is worn outside and can be emptied and changed when necessary.

A patient with an ileal conduit needs to have access to clean water and to be near a medical facility where she can obtain a regular supply of bags, and she has to have expert help if she needs it. For those reasons it's not possible for such a patient to return to her village.

Desta Mender is situated in the midst of fertile farming country outside Addis Ababa. It's a peaceful location; there's no hint that the stink and pollution of the city is only half an hour away. The original plan was that it would be a typical rural village, with *tukuls* made of mud with thatched roofs, each housing four or five women. They'd have little gardens where they would grow food and they'd do their own cooking. All very simple. AusAID gave them a grant to build it and the Australian architect who has long been associated with the hospital, Ridley Smith, was asked to produce a design. Ridley consulted closely with the staff. One of their first suggestions was to forget about traditional construction methods. Concrete blocks would be more durable than mud, and thatch has to be replaced every fifteen years and also houses vermin. The houses are plain rendered brick, painted white with tin roofs. The little settlement nestles against the foot of a hill with a green panorama spread out before it. At the lower end there's a pretty little lake. The houses are arranged in a circle with a community centre in the middle. It's a circular building like a *tukul*. Catherine's hand is obvious in the gorgeous landscaped gardens and flagged stone pathways, reminiscent of the hospital in Addis.

Catherine always hoped that Desta Mender would be partly self-sufficient. When Jock and Louise arrived, there were the beginnings of extensive vegetable gardens, a dairy, and an apple orchard. All of this was familiar stuff for Jock. He set about organising a water supply to be pumped up from the lake, installing a generator, instructing the local staff on how to fell trees safely, and getting the dairy up and running.

He noted that the people in the nearby village were always coming down with diseases such as typhus and dysentery. They were getting their drinking water from the same waterhole that the cattle used. Jock ran a pipe from his supply to the village well and turned it on for an hour in the morning and evening. The incidence of illness went right down.

There was no blueprint for how to rehabilitate patients who had endured the trauma that these women had been through. 'The girls were fresh out of the hospital,' Louise remembers. 'Most, before their operation, had been hidden away and hadn't socialised. My job was to get them feeling they were part of life again.'

There were eighteen residents to begin with. One of the first things Louise did was take them on an outing to the nearest town. 'They wouldn't get out at the shop at first. Then they all went in and bought cheap earrings and shampoos and so on and they started to feel like women again. Next time we went by in the vehicle there was a tap on my shoulder: "Can we get out at the shop?"'

Louise would take them into the market and buy clothes, and in the evenings they'd have fashion parades. She invited kids from the local school to come and mix with the girls. Some enjoyed it, but others found it upsetting, as it reminded them of the lives they'd left behind, so Jock and Louise discontinued the practice.

Jock and Louise organised a teacher to come and give the girls some basic education, and taught some of them how to work in the vegetable garden and the dairy. They proceeded by trial and error; some ideas worked and some didn't. But the one constant was the love of these two Australian farmers for their charges. 'The girls were like our family,' Louise says.

She and Jock had to go back to Australia after a year when their son's wife contracted cancer and she had no parents of her own to care for her. This is the first time they've returned to Desta Mender.

As we drive through the gates the guards recognise them and give them a big hello, wide grins all over their faces. We park the Land Rover and start to walk up the path towards the community centre. A girl with a walking frame comes towards us moving as fast as she can go. She's Tirumaid, a polio victim since she was two, with only one workable leg. As if her life were not tragic enough, she was raped and her pregnancy caused a fistula. When she came to the hospital she was only able to crawl. Now they've got her up and walking. She proudly tells Louise and Jock that she's learning how to knit – a skill with which one day she may be able to earn a living.

Tirumaid is hanging onto Louise as if she never wants to let her go. Then another girl, Minte, comes running down the path. There are more hugs and kisses while Louise tries out her rusty Amharic. Minte leads her by the hand to her house and shows her an embroidered pillowcase she's making. Others gather round smiling and laughing.

Catherine's vision was for Desta Mender to be a home for life. But, like everything else at the Fistula Hospital, that is changing. There are now more than 50 women residents, and at the rate they're going the place will soon be full. Each person costs 33,000 to 34,000 birr per year to keep. That's about $4000 – an astronomical amount compared with the average cost of care for a fistula patient.

The idea now is to train the women how to look after their

stomas, teach them a skill they can use in the outside world, then help them set up little businesses. They could return to their own language and tribal areas and be near one of the new outreach hospitals if assistance were needed. Three are functioning already and another two are being built. When the hospitals are completed they will cover the northern, southern, eastern and western parts of the country. So, Desta Mender will become more of a way station on the path to a new life than a permanent home.

As we move along the flower-bordered paths it's like a triumphal procession, with girls coming up to say hello, squeals of recognition, excited questions and answers, and plenty of smiles and laughter. At the dairy we encounter a Muslim girl, Ajebush, wearing a pretty headscarf. I have a vivid memory of Ajebush from my previous visit. Even as one of many tragic cases, hers was unforgettable. Dr Ambaye, one of the hospital's long-serving doctors, had found Ajebush on one of her outreach trips. She had been operating at the hospital in Metu in the west of the country, when they told her about a girl with a fistula who'd been lying in a hut in a village for years. When Ambaye walked into the hut the smell was so bad that she almost vomited. Ajebush had been lying on a goatskin bed in a room with one small window for nine years, never seeing the sun. Her only human contact was with her sister, who brought her food. Because of the darkened room and her poor diet, the calcium in her bones had leached away. Lying on her side, her hip bones had collapsed into the middle. Ambaye brought her back to Addis. It took three years to get Ajebush walking.

When I met Ajebush she'd been convalescing after an ileal conduit operation and had begun walking with the aid of two sticks. Because she had been isolated since the age of about fifteen, she spoke in a tiny little squeak. It was a miracle that she was alive.

Louise recalls that when they put the girls into house groups and they started cooking their own meals, Ajebush quickly showed that she was a leader. She was one of the brightest girls there. She started going to school and was first in her class when she graduated from grade two. She's currently in elementary school; she could even go on to higher education. She has a job looking after the records in the dairy and keeps them better than the hired staff used to do. Soon they're going to ask her to keep the accounts as well.

Last year Ajebush was well enough to return home to her village for a visit. It was the first time she'd been back in nine years. She put on a new white dress for the big occasion. When a woman saw her walking up the path to the village she fled in terror. She thought it was Ajebush's ghost come back to haunt them.

Louise asks her about the future. 'Well, I know who I was,' she replies. 'It's after I came here that I became somebody. I will be happy to do any work that you give me.'

Ajebush still has serious disabilities. She has days when her back hurts so badly that she can't move. But the twice-daily walk to the dairy is making her stronger. Before, she was painfully shy; her confidence is growing all the time.

We are introduced to a tall, graceful lady and her five-year-old daughter. In contrast to the other girls, Habite's demeanour is very grave. And when you hear her story you can understand why. In her village there was a *wogesha* who was treating piles with battery acid. He put so much of it into Habite that it created a huge rectal fistula. It's a strange thought, but maybe she was lucky. The next person the *wogesha* treated died.

The only thing they could do for Habite was give her a colostomy bag. She's here convalescing from the operation and learning how to manage her condition. Habite used to work in the former French colony Djibouti as a housemaid. She's had some education and can speak French. Her daughter, Rachel, is the only child at Desta Mender and needs to be where she can go to school and be with other children. They're going to try to get Habite a job with one of the staff from the French Embassy in Addis.

Our guide is the manager, Ephraim Aklilu, a gentle, softly spoken man of about 30. He's an agriculturalist. At university he majored in plant science and minored in animal husbandry. He taught in a few different agricultural colleges then he worked at the Carter Centre for Peace and Democracy, which was set up by the former American president to observe the 2005 elections.

Ephraim likes to help people. When he heard they were looking for staff at Desta Mender he thought that here was the opportunity he had been seeking.

He'd already heard a lot about Catherine Hamlin before he met her. 'I started here as a job, but it became more than that. Everyone knows about Dr Hamlin; everybody loves Dr Hamlin; everybody is inspired by Dr Hamlin. When we think about good people they usually share their vision and make you part of their vision. I'm now one of those people.'

Another key person at Desta Mender is an Englishwoman, Rosemary Burke. In England she spent twenty years as a high-powered business consultant buying and selling companies. While travelling during her holidays she saw how in the third world a great deal could be done with very little, and that a little bit of expertise went a long way. The idea that she should be using her skills where they could really do some good, rather than just improving some company's share price, kept niggling at her. So, she changed from working with merchant bankers and lawyers – mostly men – to working with uneducated and profoundly disabled peasant women. Rosemary is here for six months, devising suitable micro enterprises.

Silkworms are one such idea. '[The women] should be able to spin silk because most of them spin cotton, then that will provide a good income. They could keep silkworms and chickens and feed the dead worms to the chickens; combine that with a vegie patch, then you've got something. Little patches of land are quite enough for half a dozen chickens, and silkworms don't need much. We've seen urban agriculture where you plant things in bashed-out oil drums with slits in the side; you can get a good crop growing on your verandah. I want to try to get these women doing that sort of thing.'

Rosemary has organised sewing lessons for some of the residents. The first two are about to leave Desta Mender and return to their own area in the south. The hospital has bought them two sewing machines and arranged rental accommodation near the outreach hospital at Yirgalem.

No one knows exactly how these two pioneers will fare. Educated women in Ethiopia sometimes live away from their families, but uneducated women don't. How will they fit in with society? Will they be labelled as odd? Will they be subject to unwelcome attention? Rosemary says, 'These two and the next group are a bit of an experiment, just to understand what preparation we have to give them, whether this whole idea is going to work. We just don't know. It's a step into the dark.'

Mark Bennett envisages a future where patients will spend about eighteen months at Desta Mender before moving on. During that time they'll be taught how to manage their medical condition, they'll be given some basic literacy skills, and they'll be trained in a skill that they can use in the outside world. While they're at Desta Mender they can help out in the orchard or the vegetable gardens or the dairy, all of which, Mark says, can generate income for the village. There are also plans to market artemisia, an anti-malarial plant, and to produce honey. When the time comes for the women to leave, the hospital will help them set up their enterprise. Those who'd like to continue working at Desta Mender can apply for a position if there's one available. If they are employed they'll receive a wage, live outside and pay rent like any other worker. Of course those whose medical condition is so chronic they cannot leave will continue to be looked after.

'When Desta Mender was first created we didn't have the expertise or the people to make it work practically,' says Mark. 'Well, now we've just about got that and we're starting to see some of those things happen. I think that's so exciting. And when the first women leave we ought to have a great celebration and we should do everything we can to make their life a great success outside Desta Mender.'

Back at the hospital that evening there's a small dinner party at Ruth's house overlooking the river. It's often a mere trickle but this evening it's a muddy torrent; the air is filled with a roar like storm-driven surf. It hasn't rained that day, so Catherine surmises that there must have been a storm up in the hills. She reminisces about the early days when she and Richard – without Reg, as he didn't care for horses – used to ride out from the Princess Tsehai Hospital over rolling countryside dotted with little *tukuls*. Sometimes they'd cross a river, only to find when they returned a few hours later that it was in full flood. That countryside she's talking about has now been submerged by development.

Jock and Louise are with us. They're going back to Australia in a day or two. Another guest is Felicity Mussel, an English missionary doctor who works as an obstetrician in a remote part of Bangladesh. The American church which employs her has funded a fistula ward in her hospital. One surgeon has already trained in Addis and Felicity is the second. It's an indication of how aid providers have recently begun to do something about fistula in the developing world. Felicity is finding the surgery very challenging. Before she came she'd heard that Catherine was still operating. She says, 'If I hadn't seen it with my own eyes I wouldn't have believed it.'

Before we sit down to dinner we can hear a thunderstorm brewing. The lights flicker once or twice and Ruth prepares a few candles in case there's a blackout. Most of the hospital is hooked up to an emergency generator which starts automatically if the power fails, but Ruth's house is not connected.

The conversation gets around to Ethiopian food. 'What's *wat*?' Felicity wants to know.

This brings a laugh. Not at all put out, Felicity comes back with, 'I'll bet no one here knows where's Ware?'

More laughter. She's right. No one does know where Ware is. It turns out it's the name of a town in Hertfordshire. This little bit of foolishness has introduced a playful mood. 'Cath, pass me some bread, please,' says Jock.

Catherine tosses him a piece down the length of the table. Jock manages to catch it and Catherine breaks into girlish laughter. We're back in the family home at Ryde, where Catherine and Jock used to get up to all sorts of naughtiness. Once Catherine got into trouble for dropping hot potatoes from a tree onto the backs of slumbering cows. When Jock was asked why he'd done something naughty his excuse was, 'God told me to.' Such misdemeanours usually earned an appointment with their mother's hairbrush.

The after-dinner entertainment is Jock reading aloud chapter five of *Winnie-the-Pooh*. Just before he begins there's an extra loud crash of thunder and the lights really do go out.

Ruth lights the candles and we sit in a circle in her lounge room – the drawing room, as Catherine would call it – and we're entranced, as Jock, with the same precise English diction as his sister, reads about the adventures of Pooh and Piglet as they plan to trap a heffalump.

It's like being transported back to another century, before TV and blockbuster movies, e-mail and the internet. Catherine has created her own little world here. She never watches television, or listens to the radio. Information about the outside world comes to her via the weekly *Telegraph*, airmailed from London. She's frequently appalled by the news it contains, of the increasing secularism and selfishness and falling moral standards of modern society.

Jock feels the same. He preferred to travel via the Muslim-owned airline Emirates, as he's found the movies on Qantas 'quite unsuitable'. Back in Australia he stopped having his hair cut in town years ago because he suspected the hairdresser was a homosexual. Louise cuts it for him.

In the background the river roars; now and then, thunder rattles the windows and the candles flicker. When the reading ends we talk about our favourite childhood books. Enid Blyton, *Swallows and Amazons* and *Alice in Wonderland* get a mention. I feel as though I've been through the looking-glass myself, into the forgotten world of Catherine's childhood. And what a privilege that is.

A few days later I return to Desta Mender for a school graduation ceremony. Up until grade three the women are taught by a teacher who comes out every day from Addis. After grade three the women go on to night school. Nine are graduating; three have completed third year and five are going to night school. The community hall has been prepared for the occasion by grass having been scattered over the floor. For the guests there's warm Coca-Cola or Sprite, popcorn and little pieces of bread cut from a giant square loaf. The initial cuts are always made in the shape of a cross. And of course there's strong, sweet coffee in tiny cups, without which no Ethiopian ceremony would be complete.

Jock and Louise have gone home to Australia. Ephraim is at the hall as are most of the other staff. Ruth has brought along three women from Sierra Leone who are visiting Addis Ababa. One is a university professor, the other two are lecturers.

About 40 girls are sitting in chairs waiting expectantly for the speeches to begin. Most are aged in their teens up to mid-twenties. I look at these rows of beautiful dark faces and can't help feeling regret for their ruined lives. They are broken women, I'm thinking, but then I remind myself that if they weren't here they'd most likely be dead. Better to feel regret for the thousands of other women who have not had medical care, who are suffering and dying all over the country. These are the lucky ones.

The first young woman comes up to receive her certificate and a prize. Yeshalem is in her mid-twenties, I'd guess, wearing a pretty green dress, her hair braided into neat rows. She's graduating from second grade. She hobbles over with the help of a crutch. She was left at the hospital gate a few years ago, paralysed after falling out of a tree. She wasn't a fistula patient, but they took her in anyway, and cared for her, gave her physiotherapy, and now she can walk with the aid of her crutch. Her teacher, Zuriashwerke, a slim young woman with a shock of big hair, congratulates her and hands her a certificate. All the girls grin and applaud.

Zuriashwerke has been teaching here for four years. Before, she was at a kindergarten in a private school in Addis, teaching privileged kids from wealthy families. She knew nothing about fistulas or the hard life of rural women. At first she was overwhelmed by the state of the girls. They were reluctant to learn, as they couldn't see the point of it. It just wasn't part of the life they'd known. Many did not know how to keep themselves clean, or sleep in a bed or use a toilet. She wondered what she'd got herself into. But she persevered and found that once they started, the girls loved to learn. She says they're great students. There's no reason why they could not graduate from school and go to university. They all tell her their history, and every time they do, she ends up crying with them.

After Yeshalem accepts her prize she gives Zuriashwerke a present of a cane jewellery box, a *muda*, that she's made herself. One by one, the others come up and receive their certificates and bask in the applause. The students clearly adore Zuriashwerke and she adores them.

When it's over, Ruth makes a speech, Ephraim also says something, then one of the ladies from Sierra Leone gets up. With Ephraim translating, she tells the women about the importance of education. She says that with education they'll be able to care for their children properly, they'll be able to read the labels on medicine bottles, their kids will have better opportunities. The more she blunders on, the more incredulous I become. The magic of the occasion has been spoiled. These women are never going to have children, they're never going to have husbands or anything resembling a normal family life. Poor Ephraim continues to translate her nonsense without flinching. The residents listen impassively. When, mercifully, she stops talking and sits down, I wonder what on earth can be done to repair the damage.

Then Ruth gets to her feet. She tells them that when they leave Desta Mender and go back to their villages, the children of their brothers and sisters will look upon them as mothers. They'll play games with them and come to them for advice and comfort, just as if they were their own children. It will be the same, she says. It's a brilliant save. And, who knows, if the plans for this place work out as hoped and these women do one day return to their communities, what Ruth has said could turn out to be true.

CHAPTER 9

The decision to resort to an ileal conduit is only made after other operations to cure incontinence have been tried and failed or where the bladder has been destroyed during the obstructed labour. A patient may endure half a dozen surgical procedures, spread out over years, before reaching this final, drastic point. Agreeing to the operation is a life-changing decision. It means that they may not be able to live in their home village ever again and they will face a lifetime of dependence on medical help. The decision is irrevocable. A urinary diversion is not reversible.

Not all women agree to the operation. Some prefer the rejection and loneliness of their condition to the prospect of having a bag attached to their body for the rest of their lives. All the counselling in the world does not prevent them from being deeply ashamed of the bag. They see it as a stigma – so much so that the hospital staff find it almost impossible to persuade women with stomas to help teach new patients how to manage them.

When a diversion is the only option left, the person who has the sensitive task of breaking the news is Sister Ruth Gadessa. Ruth is a warm and motherly woman in her early thirties who seems always to be smiling. She is dedicated absolutely to the welfare of the damaged young women in her care. In her bright, sunny office one morning she is counselling a shy young woman from Gojjam province in the north-west. Fantaye Atabay doesn't know how old she is (Ruth guesses about 22 or 23). And she doesn't know exactly when she got married. She remembers that she went into labour on a Saturday and her child was stillborn on a Monday. She had a double fistula. Her husband left her and she went to live with her grandmother and uncle.

Fantaye has a tattooed cross at the outer corner of each eye and a tribal motif tattooed along her jawline. She speaks in a quiet little voice, eyes downcast to her lap, where her fingers worry at a loose thread in her scarf. In the last six years she has been through five operations. With the first, she had her fistulas repaired, but after rehabilitation she was still leaking urine. They sent her home and told her to come back in six months' time. Often the incontinence settles down after a few months, as the bladder and urethra begin to work normally again. Not in Fantaye's case. It took her four years to return to the hospital because she didn't have the money.

Her last operation was nine months ago. When it was obvious that it, too, had failed, Sister Ruth spoke to her about the possibility of a urinary diversion. She suggested that she go back home for a while to think about it but Fantaye had no wish to return. 'It's too hurtful to go back,' she told Ruth. 'All the time I've been having surgery I haven't wanted to see anyone. When I go back to my village I feel sad. I've lost all of my friends. Why should I go when I'm like this?'

In Addis she's been staying at Rebecca's Place, a house owned by a wealthy American philanthropist where a lot of waiting patients stay. Ruth asks if her grandmother knows how to get in touch with her. Fantaye hasn't told her grandmother where she is. She says that because of her problem everyone in her family has suffered, and she feels they've had enough of her.

'Well, you've got a friend here,' says Ruth, with an affection-ate little pat. 'I'm your friend.'

Not for the first time in this place I feel close to tears. Fantaye's life has been ruined before she's even *had* a life. The worst of it is that it's so unnecessary. In developed countries such as Australia it's a century since any woman had an obstetric fistula due to childbirth. With enough trained midwives and timely access to hospitals they could be unknown here as well.

Ruth shows Fantaye some anatomical drawings and explains to her what a urinary diversion is and how a stoma works. It's hard to tell if she really understands. Ruth thinks she does, but says it's difficult for women who've never had any education to comprehend the explanation.

Ruth puts a stoma bag on the desk and shows it to her. Fantaye eyes it warily without touching it. She doesn't say anything.

Ruth then tells her that nearly all the nurse aides at the hospital – about 70 women – have ileal conduits. Fantaye is interested in that. She's seen the nurse aides in their clean, pressed uniforms working around the wards. They seem happy and normal. She thought all the ileal conduit cases were at Desta Mender. No, Ruth tells her, there are lots here and in the other centres as well.

Then she puts on an American-made video, with animation showing how a diversion works. There are testimonies from Americans with stomas who have been living normal lives for years. Fantaye is amazed that men have them too. 'Are you telling me the truth?' she asks.

'Yes, it's not only because of birth injuries; there are other causes.'

When the video ends, Fantaye asks a series of questions. She's stopped fiddling with her shawl and is looking directly at Ruth when she speaks. I'm amazed at the difference in her demeanour. It's as if suddenly she's realised there's hope. Ruth tells her if she has the operation she will have to go to Desta Mender for a while. She'll need to be a good student and learn a skill well, so that she can decide what she wants to do with her future.

After a bit more conversation Fantaye decides. 'I think I'd better have it, because I don't want to go home like this. If I'm going to be okay, then let anything be done for me.'

Now that she's made up her mind she actually seems cheerful. I expected floods of tears, anger maybe, or a plunge into depression, but what I'm seeing is quiet acceptance. It's that fatalism again. Fantaye will move out of Rebecca's Place and stay at the hospital until a urologist from Britain, Gordon Williams, makes one of his regular visits to do the operation.

CHAPTER 10

The nurse aides used to all live within the compound. When their numbers grew so that there was no more room, there was a lot of discussion about moving them into outside accommodation. Catherine, who looks upon every one of them as one of her children, was very worried. 'They're going to be raped and abused,' she said. Thankfully, Catherine's fears proved unfounded; the new arrangement has worked out fine. Some still live in the compound; others are scattered around in rental accommodation.

One day Catherine, Ruth Kennedy and I go to visit some girls who live in a big old house that the hospital rents for them a couple of kilometres away. It's owned by an Ethiopian man who lives in America.

There's a big lounge room and three bedrooms, with single beds to accommodate fifteen to twenty people. In typical Ethiopian fashion the toilets are in a separate building outside, and the cooking is done in another separate little shed.

When we arrive, one of the girls, Bossena, is sitting on the couch in the lounge room with two friends visiting from her village. It's the first time that they've been to Addis Ababa.

They're watching a cheesy Ethiopian television drama with rapt expressions on their faces. They've never seen TV before.

When we come in, the girls move to another couch so as to give us the honoured place in front of the TV. Catherine has told the girls not to do anything special for us, but she knows that they will anyway. They offer us some bread and popcorn and warm soft drink. They've prepared some *injera* and a *wat* of stewed goat.

A tall, slim young woman comes into the room. Catherine's face lights up when she sees her. She introduces her as Wokinesh and pats the seat beside her. 'Come and sit here, darling.' Wokinesh sits down, Catherine puts her arm around her and she snuggles against her with a happy smile. Wokinesh is one of Catherine's favourites. They have quite a history together. She was eighteen when she came to the hospital with terrible injuries. She had two fistulas and severe contractures of her limbs. Her hair was rust-coloured, which is a sign of malnutrition. 'She was moribund,' says Catherine. 'She was really dying. She was so weak she couldn't lift herself up from the bed. She came to us less than a month after delivery, totally septic, completely infected. The conditions she'd been living under must have been awful. Her family had just given up on her.'

They shaved her hair, fed her good, nourishing food, and gave her physiotherapy. When she was strong enough they repaired her fistulas. Then she had to have her gall bladder removed. After eighteen months at the hospital she was dry and they were ready to send her home. 'She'd just been a little skeleton lying in the bed,' Catherine recalls. 'She was risen from the dead.'

Catherine was so impressed with her spirit that when Wokinesh asked if she could be a nurse aide she said yes. 'She's very good,' says Catherine, for all the world like a proud mother. 'She knows everything about every patient in the ward.'

A smiling young woman, Fatuma, comes in and sits down

beside Bossena. Fatuma is wearing a headscarf. They're both from Gonder in the north-west, one an Orthodox Christian, the other a Muslim. When Bossena had her operation she went into a deep depression. She'd curl up in bed and refuse to speak, or else she'd go wandering off and try to harm herself. One time they found her up in a tree in the compound. Andrew Browning had to go up and bring her down.

When Fatuma arrived at the hospital she, too, was suffering from severe depression. Ruth remembers that her eyes were dead. 'She was completely switched off. She didn't speak for six months.'

After a lot of counselling and anti-depressant medication, Bossena started speaking and she had her operation. Then, when Fatuma began to improve, they thought that she was ready for *her* operation. Close examination revealed that there was nothing to work with, her anatomy was a total ruin. So Matron Edjigayehu and Sister Ruth Gadissa sat her down and told her, 'You're going to have to have an operation and you're not going to be able to go back to your village. It's going to be an opening on the abdomen and you'll have to wear a bag.'

Fatuma looked at them and said, 'Does that mean I get to be a nurse aide?'

Matron said, 'Would you like that?'

'More than anything.'

'Then you can be a nurse aide.'

'Then please do the operation.'

Some time later Ruth went into the ward and heard riotous giggling. Bossena and Fatuma, both about seventeen, were in bed together laughing like a couple of schoolgirls.

'What are you doing?' said Ruth. They just giggled some more.

When Fatuma got her nurse aide's uniform Bossena slipped back into depression. One day Matron found her lying in bed with her face to the wall. 'Bossy, what's the matter?'

'You gave Fatuma a uniform. What about me?'

'Do you want a uniform?'

'Of course.'

So they gave Bossena a uniform, and neither she nor Fatuma have shown a sign of depression since. Bossena could probably go home if she wanted to, but Matron says that if she were to send her away it would destroy Fatuma. You can't separate them. They're kindred spirits.

It's time to check on my patients whom I've been tracking. You see, I think of them as 'my patients' now. Amina is sitting up in bed looking a lot happier than when I last saw her. It was a couple of days after her operation and she was hungry and sore. Now on her fourth post-operative day she's back on her normal diet of *injera* and *wat*, of which Ethiopians never seem to tire. She has a catheter and so far her rehabilitation is progressing well – dry, drinking and draining, as the doctors like to say. That is, there's no leaking from a breakdown in the fistula repair, she's drinking enough to keep up a good urine output to irrigate the healing bladder, and the catheter is not blocked, so her bladder won't fill and burst the repair.

Amina is an open, outgoing young woman. Her expressive eyes reveal every emotion and she's happy to answer all of my questions. I think it makes her feel special that the *ferenji* is taking such an interest in her. She's been thinking about her future: she definitely doesn't want another husband. When she goes home she'd like to go to school. The reality is that neither of these wishes is likely to come true.

Dr Abiy's patient, Zemebech, is also progressing well. She's dry, drinking and draining too. Abiy is at her bedside when I drop by, and both doctor and patient are pleased with her progress. Abiy has a sympathetic bedside manner. He treats the patients with respect and they respond gratefully to his concern. He says he has 90 per cent decided on a career in fistula surgery, but it will depend on some negotiations with the Ministry of Health. Every medical student has to spend a certain time in country hospitals after they graduate and he's hoping that the time he's spent in postgraduate study at Jimma may count.

Later when I see Catherine I tell her what Abiy has said. 'That's good,' she says, 'but of course they often change their minds.'

Halema, the Somali patient, gives me a wan look when I see her. I can't read much into it. There's no one there to translate, but Dr Biruk, who operated on her four days ago, says she's doing well. She's also d, d and d.

Alganish, the lady from Tigray who's worried about her children being neglected, has had her surgery. She gives me a big smile, revealing a row of white teeth with generous gaps between them. The medical director, Dr Mulu, did her operation. She says the fistula in the rectum was not difficult, but there is concern about Alganish's bladder. Mulu lengthened the urethra and changed the angle by using a supporting 'sling' of muscle. It's quite likely that although her fistulas have been cured, Alganish will suffer from stress incontinence. Because they reconstructed the urethra they're going to leave the catheter in for three weeks rather than two, to give a better chance of healing.

Alganish looks happy. She says that she's grateful for the care that she's getting. Although because of the language barriers I can't converse directly with these patients, I feel I'm beginning to glean some understanding of their different personalities.

I suspect that Alganish will always be positive, no matter how many hard knocks life throws at her.

Leteabazgi, the girl whose soldier friend brought her down from Tigray, had her operation yesterday. She's in the recovery section of the ward and is feeling pretty awful. She's nauseous and not really up to talking.

Dr Habte's patient, Letelibanes, is doing well. She's feeling happy about life. Her son is safe at home with her mother and father, so she isn't worried about him. She's looking forward to going home cured and to a new life, helping her parents out on their farm.

CHAPTER 11

In the year 2000 when I was working with Catherine on her biography, her greatest concern was for the future of the hospital after she'd gone. They were never desperately short of money, but at the same time they never had quite enough to invest for the future. While Reg had been alive he'd done most of the fund-raising. After he died, Catherine doubted she'd have the same ability but she has proved to be just as adept as her husband was. Maybe even better. Her grace and charm, and obvious goodness, can melt the hardest heart. Former Australian Foreign Minister Gareth Evans once told her, 'You're my favourite pin-up girl; how can I help?' The result of that conversation was a million-dollar capital works program to upgrade the hospital, funded by AusAID.

Although she's remarkably good at raising money, Catherine can be vague about the details. 'Mr Downer the [then current Australian] foreign minister has given me a lot of money, two million Australian dollars. I went to see him when I was in Canberra last. I don't know how we got the first million but it was from him through AusAID. He said to me, "What are you going to do now that you've got this two million?"

'"Well", I said, "we'll just go on begging."

'He laughed; I think he's very keen.'

Reg and Catherine have had numerous honours bestowed upon them by medical bodies and universities. Reg was awarded an OBE by the Queen; the Australian government made Catherine a Companion of the Order of Australia, she's been nominated for the Nobel Peace Prize, she's been awarded the Rotary International Award for World Understanding. Despite all of this recognition and the goodwill of the Australian government, the desperate need of fistula sufferers remained largely ignored by the rest of the world until recently.

The year that *The Hospital by the River* was published, things began to change. This wasn't just because of the book, although it did help. From about 2001 onwards, large aid providers began to show an interest. Dr Ambaye had been making regular trips to regional government hospitals for years to operate on fistula patients. Suddenly Columbia University's Averting Maternal Death and Disability (AMDD) program was asking if there was anything they could do to help. AMDD bought new operating tables and theatre lights for four hospitals. Some doctors in Oxford, England, put instrument kits together. In 2002 the United Nations Population Fund (UNFPA) decided to begin a global campaign with a budget of $75 million to end obstetric fistula. UNFPA, the American government aid agency USAID (United States Agency for International Development), and others were asking if they could contribute to the hospital. At the same time, donations to the various trusts in the UK, Europe, America and Australia were on the increase.

In 2004 Catherine and Ruth made a trip to inspect the outreach centres in government hospitals, with a view to upgrading some of the facilities. When they returned to Addis they and the trustees discussed building a couple of new wards and such things as improving kitchen facilities. It meant spending

$100,000 here, $60,000 there. When they thought about it some more, they decided that rather than patch up what was there they might be better off building new fistula hospitals. Plans were made to build five small hospitals to cover the northern, southern, eastern and western regions of the country.

And then there was Oprah.

The head of the US trust in the early part of 2000, Ric Haas, had been trying for a couple of years to get Catherine a spot on *The Oprah Winfrey Show*. A few minutes with America's talk show queen has been known instantly to change the fortunes of her guests. Books by obscure authors suddenly become bestsellers; struggling charities find themselves swamped with donations. Oprah's show is watched by 49 million viewers each week in the United States, and millions more in 117 other countries. No wonder Ric was trying hard.

In the end, though, it was a friend of Catherine's, Deborah Harris, who lives in Georgia, USA, who pulled it off. Deborah's husband, John, knew people on Oprah's production team, and in January 2004, Catherine was invited to go to Chicago to be interviewed before a studio audience.

In the hotel the day before they were due to meet Oprah, Catherine asked Ruth, 'How will we know who she is? Do you know what she looks like?'

Ruth had to admit she had no idea. She hurriedly bought a copy of *O Magazine* which had a picture of Oprah on the cover, so that solved that problem.

On the appointed day they were driven to the studio in a limousine. When they walked into the green room there was no doubt about who Oprah was.

'How do you do, Miss Winfrey,' said Catherine.

Oprah laughed. 'No, no,' she said. 'Don't call me Miss Winfrey. Everybody calls me Oprah.'

They were an unlikely pair. The loud, extrovert, billionaire entertainer, who had risen from dirt-poor beginnings to host the highest-rating TV talk show in syndication history, and the refined, conservative, missionary doctor, who had spent most of her life quietly going about her life-saving medical work in Ethiopia. Oprah and Catherine hit it off immediately.

They began the segment with some sequences filmed in Ethiopia that explained fistulas. There were some moving scenes of Dr Ambaye on one of her outreach trips discovering women who'd been living in isolation for many years. They profiled two cases, Hawa and Majo. Hawa had borne six children, only one of whom had lived. Her last child had been stillborn. When Ambaye found her she had been living with a fistula for twenty years.

The camera showed Ambaye sitting in the dim hut where Hawa lived. Ambaye told her they could do an operation that would mend the hole completely. 'Would you like that?' she asked.

'I would be so happy to visit people again,' said Hawa. As the camera held tight on her lined and careworn face, tears welled in her eyes.

Oprah's audience gasped when they heard how the next case, Majo, had been betrothed at the age of eight. The studio camera showed shocked looks on their faces as they were confronted with the reality of women's lives in less fortunate countries than their own.

Majo told how she had been in labour for six days before her child was born dead. 'I can't hold my head up,' she said. 'There's nothing I can do about it.'

Both Hawa and Majo had been cured. There was a pre-recorded message from Mamitu thanking Catherine for everything she'd done for her. Then came the interview.

I've seen Catherine speak to audiences many times, and the

reaction is always the same. She speaks quietly, as if she were holding a normal conversation. No dramatics or staged pauses or exaggerated gestures. But the story she has to tell is so powerful that within a few moments listeners become totally absorbed. It was no different with Oprah's American audience. The camera now and then cut away to show rapt faces, mouths open in shock, streaming tears. Even Oprah was subdued.

'How are you funded?' she asked.

'We beg. My husband and I always used to say we're professional beggars.'

The matter-of-fact way in which this was delivered brought an uneasy laugh from the audience. The show was a bit more the style they were used to when, a little later, Catherine commented that if fistula were a men's problem something would have been done about it years ago.

Oprah: 'If a man had a hole in his penis? You're darn right about that! Even the men here would know that, do you think?' The camera cut away to show sheepish male faces. 'If there was a problem with men with a hole in their penises there'd be a Hole in the Penis Committee immediately to fix that.'

'Oprah was nice,' says Catherine. 'She just asked me questions. She had a film going in the background showing some of the women. There were lots of ladies crying in the audience. Reg used to say unless they cry I don't think we've done any good. It's a very appealing thing to talk about, I think, especially for women.'

When the show ended, Oprah asked Catherine to come up to her office, something she rarely does with guests. During the interview Oprah had asked, 'How much does it cost to run the hospital for a year?'

'About 450,000 dollars US.'

In the office Oprah got out her personal chequebook and wrote out a cheque for $450,000.

After recovering from her surprise, Catherine thanked her warmly. 'Why don't you come and see our work?' she said.

'I will come,' replied Oprah.

After consultation with the US trustees it was decided to use part of Oprah's donation to build a new wing to house a urodynamics department, Sister Ruth Gadessa's stomal therapy unit and a teaching centre for nurse aides. By the time the promised visit was due, the building was not quite finished, but there was enough of a structure for Oprah to perform the opening ceremony.

The visit was arranged for December 2004, when Oprah was on her way to South Africa to see about a new girls' school she was building with her own money. An advance party of three producers came to Addis to discuss the arrangements with Ruth Kennedy, who is in charge of media matters. One of them asked if it would be all right for Oprah to give the girls dresses. She told him it would be fine as long as they were long ones with sleeves. They were glad they'd asked. They'd been planning on giving them little string-sleeved tops and miniskirts. The skirts were acceptable, as Ethiopian women wear them like that with trousers underneath, but the skimpy tops would have been an embarrassing mistake.

Oprah specifically requested that the visit be kept low key, with no press and no dignitaries. She just wanted to meet Catherine, her staff and the patients. There would be no problem keeping the press out as the compound is completely surrounded by high walls with guarded gates. But the second request created a dilemma, as the land on which the new wing had been built had been given to them on a free 99-year lease by the Mayor of Addis Ababa. Catherine had a word to her new friend. 'I said to her, "Look, I have to let the mayor know you're coming because he's given me this land where we've built your centre."

'So she said, "That'll be all right if I meet him." He had a very pretty wife, she came with him. A sweet girl from Tigray.'

On the big day Oprah flew in on her private jet with a large retinue of producers and camera crews. With her were two of her viewers who, after seeing the interview with Catherine, had been inspired to help women in Africa.

Cyrene Wright, a young, African American medical student, had e-mailed every hospital in Kenya, then raised $2000 to go on an eight-week medical mission. She told Oprah, 'Dr Hamlin showed me the power of being ready to use the tools that you're given.'

Sue Hoese, a mother of two young children, had never heard of fistulas. For weeks after the interview she had been haunted by the plight of the fistula victims. One image in particular had stayed with her – of Catherine giving out new dresses to cured patients waiting to go home. Sue was struck by how important it was to give them some of their dignity back. After thinking hard, she had come up with the idea of giving each patient at the hospital a bracelet. She hosted bracelet-making meetings at her home. Sixty volunteers had made 1600 bracelets, which she had brought with her.

Oprah and her crew travelled from the airport to the hospital amidst a cavalcade of police motorcycles. They pulled up outside and Oprah got out and walked through the gate to where Catherine and a line of staff members were waiting. She threw her arms wide in greeting and announced, 'Hello, everyone!'

Catherine stepped forward to welcome her. 'I never thought you'd come.'

'I told you I was coming, and I know you didn't believe me.'

Oprah went along the line shaking hands. The mayor's wife presented her with a beautiful Ethiopian outfit which she insisted on wearing immediately. Having nowhere handy to change, she popped into the physiotherapy department. There were no curtains on the window so Ruth had to stand holding up a towel to prevent the caterers, preparing tables on the lawn, from peering in at her while she undressed.

They set off on a tour of the compound. At times Catherine lost sight of her guest as the crowd surged along from ward to ward. The film of the visit, which was broadcast after she returned home, showed Oprah visiting patients and listening to their stories. One little girl had been married at nine. Still in her teens she had had two stillborn babies and had been twice to the hospital to have fistulas repaired. She told Oprah, 'I'm not going to try for a third.'

Another patient had been raped at thirteen and ended up with a double fistula. 'I've been leaking for four years now,' she told Oprah. 'I'll be happy when I can go home cured.'

Next came a tiny little girl who looked as though she should be in school or playing with her toys. One of the nurses told Oprah that she did not speak and barely ate anything for six months. She had had her operation and was on the way to recovery.

Catherine introduced Oprah to some patients, who, in their new dresses from the hospital, were about to go home. Then it was on to some nurse aides. Mahoubar had been orphaned at the age of seven and her relatives had sold her into virtual slavery. At fifteen she was raped. When she was seven months pregnant she ran away and returned to her relatives. Far from being sympathetic, they had forced her to work in the fields until her labour began. She told Oprah that she had started labour one Wednesday and then another Wednesday passed. On Saturday the baby was born, dead of course. Mahoubar was left with a double fistula.

She was sent to live alone in an isolated hut with an open doorway. Soon hyenas, attracted by the smell of her condition, began to hang around. Mahoubar was so afraid that she crawled for a day to a mission clinic and was then brought to the hospital.

Another case – of a 37-year-old woman who had borne ten dead babies, the last one giving her a fistula. Oprah listened respectfully to each story, saying little.

She carried two baskets with her. The big one contained the dresses and the smaller had Sue's bracelets, and a collection of little purses. Oprah gave each patient a dress, a bracelet, and a purse; the purse contained makeup and lipstick and the equivalent of US$100 – more than most of the patients would earn in a year.

She showed some of the women how to use the makeup. One of the most touching images was of a patient with a look of shy delight tentatively brushing colour onto her lips, clearly for the first time in her life.

Cyrene Wright later commented that the thing which impressed her most about the visit was the smiles. 'They were a universal language for us.' For Sue it was a patient who, in thanking her for her bracelet, told her that she had 'God's heart'.

'I just wanted to let them know that I loved them and that other women across the world cared about them.'

It was just as well the press had been excluded, for if the story of the money had got out, the girls would quite likely have been mugged at the bus station on their way home. The hospital put the money into safekeeping until each one was ready to leave; and they kept quiet about it – not even the international partners knew until the TV segment was broadcast months later. To the hospital's knowledge, there were no mishaps. Oprah's generous gift must have empowered those women in a way they had never known before.

She spent a long time chatting to patients, clearly enjoying the experience. Then it was off to the new wing to declare the Oprah Winfrey Centre open.

Her only other engagement was a mayoral reception at the town hall. When she got back to her plane it had a flat tyre, so she had to spend a night at the Sheraton Hotel before continuing on to South Africa.

It had been, in Catherine's words, 'a lovely day'.

Following Catherine's interview with Oprah, her viewers had donated US$3 million to the hospital to add to Oprah's $450,000. The head of the US trust, Kate Grant, assumed that people would donate once and then move on. But that has not been the case. Donations in the following two years have reached almost $2.5 million.

While Oprah has raised millions, at the other end of the scale there are countless people of modest means, even old-age pensioners, who put aside a few dollars each week for the Fistula Hospital. In Australia, an organisation called 'Mums Kick' trains ordinary women to go mountain-climbing for charity. In 2005, fifteen women, all of them mothers – one the mother of ten – climbed Mount Kilimanjaro in Tanzania. They raised $70,000 for the new hospital at Mekele.

While Desta Mender was being built, a program about it was shown on Australian television. After the broadcast Stuart Abrahams, the retired clergyman who runs the Australian trust, received a phone call from a man in South Australia. He'd seen the show and wondered how much they needed to finish building. 'About $200,000,' said Stuart.

The money arrived shortly afterwards.

Each year Abbotsleigh Girls' School in Sydney has a service project. In 2004 it was the Fistula Hospital. They called their campaign 'To Ethiopia with Love'. The girls had three aims – to raise awareness, to donate funds and to perform some sort of practical service.

They organised an 'Ethiopian Carnival Day'. Year Twelve students manned stalls and organised such money-making activities as sponge-throwing contests, jewellery-making and face-painting. Many of the students had been so moved by what was happening to young women of their age in Ethiopia that they contributed money from their own pockets. Over a year the project raised $23,000. On the practical side, the students knitted 85 gaily-coloured woollen shawls for the patients. The Ethiopians love them; when you visit the hospital today you see the shawls everywhere.

In America, the Fistula Foundation has a program called 'Circle of Friends' which gives people the tools to host their own fund-raising events. In 2005 a group of high school girls from the Spence School in New York City organised a mother–daughter fashion show. They called it 'Girls' Night Out'. They were able to auction a number of designer dresses. The event raised $120,000.

In 2006 a supporter named Madeline McGriff organised a photography exhibition in Berkeley, California, showing pictures taken by a talented amateur photographer at the Fistula Hospital. The exhibition raised $6000.

Later in the same year Lisa Calagiovanni, a 'stay-at-home mum' from Chappaqua, New York State, raised $24,000 at an auction of donated paintings.

The US trust has a program involving expatriate Ethiopians, called Tesfa Ineste. In Amharic it means, 'Give Them Hope'. Over three years the Washington DC branch has raised $250,000 towards the new hospital at Harar.

In Britain, supporters often make use of an organisation called 'Just Giving'. Potential donors let their friends know that they have registered to support the UK fistula trust, the Hamlin Churchill Childbirth Injuries Fund. All donations, often relatively small amounts, can be channelled through this organisation. The donor does not have the hassle of dealing with hundreds of donations, and neither does the fund. According to trustee Clive Hewitt, many thousands of pounds have been raised in this way.

In mid-2005 the first of the new fistula hospitals opened at Bahar Dar in the north. The building was donated by Mr Adolfo Varnero, in memory of his father, Alberto, as a gift to the women of Ethiopia. The Varnero company has a long association with the hospital. They constructed most of the buildings in the Addis compound and built the entire complex at Desta Mender. USAID agreed to meet the running costs at Bahar Dar and also funded a project to identify fistula patients in the community.

At the beginning of 2006 a second hospital opened at Mekele in the north-east, funded by the Australian government and the Australian trust, Hamlin Fistula Relief and Aid Fund.

In November the same year a third hospital opened at Yirgalem in the south. It was funded by the Norwegian government; all the equipment was purchased by Women's Hope International, based in Switzerland. The UK fistula trust has guaranteed to cover the running costs.

At the time of writing, the new hospital at Harar in the east is three months away from opening, with funding and ongoing running costs being met by Ethiopians living in the US.

Plans for the new hospital at Metu in the west have begun. This hospital is being funded by a consortium of partners in Switzerland and the Netherlands.

As well as all these capital works, planning for a midwifery school is in the final stages. Ninety-five per cent of women who give birth in Ethiopia do so without qualified medical assistance. The problem of obstetric fistula will only ever be solved if there are trained people to help with difficult births. Catherine has been telling the government this for more than four decades, yet there are still only about a thousand midwives in all of Ethiopia, for a population of 78 million people. Just as she and Reg did back in 1959 when they saw their first fistula cases, Catherine has decided that if something is going to be done about it, she'll have to do it herself. And at last she can afford to.

CHAPTER 12

Morning prayers. Catherine, Ruth, Sister Azeb, Felicity from Bangladesh, Matron Edjigayehu, Rosemary Burke and half a dozen other regulars are here, still trudging gamely through Daniel and his prophecies.

Today there are prayers for Sister Tsedu. The oncologist in South Africa has told her that her cancer is inoperable. She's come home to Addis Ababa to undergo chemotherapy and radiation therapy. It doesn't sound good. Everyone looks solemn; Matron Edjigayehu is in tears.

There are prayers, too, for a little girl called Sayed. Sayed is in Holland recovering from heart surgery. Sayed is eleven. She's from Tigray province. After both her parents died, she was living with an elderly relative who had grown too weak to look after her. About a year ago a missionary friend of Ruth's, Karin van den Bosch, who runs a children's home, Grace Village, took her in. She noticed that whenever Sayed ran around she'd get very tired and would have to lie down to recover. Karin sent her down to Addis and asked Ruth to look after her while she had tests with a paediatric heart specialist. He diagnosed defects in the valves that go from the upper to the lower chambers on both sides of the heart, probably due to rheumatic fever as a child. Sayed needed surgery which was not available in Ethiopia.

An organisation in Holland which raises funds for Karin's children's home found a surgeon who was willing to perform the operation. Sayed came to stay with Ruth in Addis while they arranged for a passport and got permission for her to leave the country. Catherine and Ruth got to know Sayed well. One of her most memorable days was when they took her to a day of celebrations at Desta Mender. She played musical chairs with Mark Bennett's children and rode a horse, and just for a day had the sort of fun that kids in the west take for granted. Sayed called Ruth 'Sister'. Ruth remembers going to say goodnight and finding her kneeling beside her bed saying her prayers. She was saying, 'Dear God, you know I have no mother or father so you're my father and Sister's my mother.'

'She was so brave,' says Ruth. 'When she got ready to go to the Netherlands there were no tears. She stayed with a family in Holland. After she'd been there about a month, the children from the village phoned her; when she heard their voices that was the one time she broke down.'

While Sayed was having the operation, something went wrong with the oxygen machine and too much oxygen went to her brain. They don't yet know what damage has been done.

Sister Tsedu and little Sayed: that's who today's prayers are for.

A lot of prayer goes on at the hospital. Catherine's faith is the guiding light by which she lives. She begins each day with quiet prayer alone and a reading from a little book of Bible verses, the *Daily Light*. This has been her habit from when she was a schoolgirl. She believes in the power of prayer and that God's hand is in the success that the hospital has enjoyed.

She worries that as the hospital expands it may lose the Christian spirit that has guided it so far. It's not something that can be formalised in a written charter. It's an indefinable way of doing things – a Christ-like approach, if you like – that is a reflection of Catherine Hamlin's entire approach to life. She thinks it's the most important resource they have.

'We must say that we're a Christian organisation here, John. That's why we've prospered. God has been behind the work. He's the one that's been sustaining all these trusts and so on. I'm sure it's because of God that we've prospered. We must keep Him at the head of our work and must remain nominally Christian, at any rate. We're not a mission hospital. We have Muslims on the staff. But we don't want to forget that. That's really important in our charter – that we're trying to show our Lord's compassion for these people.'

Patients can attend Bible lessons at the hospital if they wish, or they can view a dramatised video in several different languages about the story of Jesus. Catherine says they have these resources because the patients think they've been cursed by God. 'We want them to know that God loves them,' she says. No one coerces the patients; it's entirely voluntary. And no one is ever refused admission because of their religion or lack of it.

One of the staff who is a Protestant has given up coming to morning prayers because some of the worshippers are Orthodox. 'That's terrible,' says Catherine. 'I said to her, "How could you do such a thing?"'

'Biruk's a keen Christian. Haile's a keen Orthodox Christian with a true faith, and so is his wife. Matron is Orthodox. Mulu is Orthodox. They're purely Christians. They trust our Lord and they trust God and they pray and they read His word. Just because they have a different way of worshipping doesn't mean they're not Christians.'

If that staff list sounds like an overload of believers, it's important to remember that in Ethiopia it's uncommon *not* to have faith, either Christian or Muslim – the opposite of the situation in the west. Unlike people in the developed world – perhaps the majority there – the average Ethiopian regards religious faith as a given. They talk about God or Allah without embarrassment. It's not at all unusual for the staff members to pray with one another about their work. It seems a natural thing to do. It's not religious zealotry; faith is just the underpinning for everything they do.

Everyone at morning prayers follows the readings in their Bibles – except for Mark Bennett, who has the Old and the New testaments downloaded onto his PalmPilot. This says something about Mark. He's the modern business expert brought in to steer the Fistula Hospital through the changes that are happening. He certainly has the credentials. He spent ten years at Arnott's Biscuits in Sydney as the manufacturing manager. Soon after he started working there, he began to wonder if this was where his future really lay. After three years he joined the senior management superannuation fund. They gave him a document showing his retirement date as 26 May 2025. He thought to himself, Is this where I'm going to be in 2025?

He'd been with Arnott's for about eight years when he married Annette, who's a trained midwife. They are both dedicated Christians. When they talked about their future they decided that making biscuits wasn't really their goal in life. They wanted to do missionary work overseas.

When Mark's general manager asked him why he was resigning he told him he wanted to study theology and work as a missionary. Normally when a senior executive resigns they tell them to leave immediately, as they don't want them taking information to competitors. Instead, Mark's boss said, 'How can we help you?'

He suggested to Mark that he keep the company car and work whatever hours he could fit in. That would justify the car, and he'd have a bit of pocket money as well. With his long-service leave and annual leave owing, and eight hours a week at Arnott's, he had enough money to see him through a year of theological college.

Mark's first missionary assignment was with the Church Missionary Society (CMS) in Egypt. He worked for eight years with the CMS helping Sudanese refugees to settle. Then he put in another two years as a development consultant with them. Mark and Annette had two children when they went to Egypt, and two more while they were there.

After ten years they thought it was time to look around for a new challenge. They would have liked to keep working in the region, but for a family with four children, it wasn't easy to find the right opportunity. They were about to go back to Australia, with no plans in place, when they heard that the Fistula Hospital was looking for a CEO.

'When I first came I was overwhelmed with what an amazing place the hospital was and what a privilege it was to work here,' Mark says. 'I couldn't believe the opportunity. In some respects the place is blessed with so many good things. No organisation I've worked with has been so well resourced, well supported and well run by everyone. It is going through a process of rapid growth. There are lots of new centres and new things they need to be doing. The marketplace they work in is changing.'

Marketplace? Mark still sometimes slips into corporate-speak. And he carries with him the competitive instincts that he learnt in the harsh secular world of business.

'The Hamlins have been here for 40 years or longer, doing fistula surgery, and for most of that time nobody else was interested. In the last five years or so there's been more international interest in the problem. Larger organisations are now focusing on it. The Hamlins were the pioneers and were the authority; now lots of others are claiming authority and looking for funds. We're

resting on 40 years of experience and expertise, but there are
other players now who are looking for the same funds. We have
to maintain our position as the leader.'

Catherine and Reg ran the hospital pretty much like a family
business. They didn't need sophisticated accounting systems; they
made the decisions and a board of trustees invariably approved
them. If one of the staff had a problem they talked about it and
sorted it out. It was pretty straightforward, but that really doesn't
work anymore for an organisation that employs more than 200
people.

Mark has proposed some changes – from salaries, to financial
systems, to the management structure. One of his proposals is to
have heads of department. For instance, the head of the Medical
Department would have the authority and accountability to run
that department. He or she would report to him and in turn
he'd keep the trustees informed about how the department was
running.

Mark's proposal is the accepted model for most similar organisations, but the senior staff at the hospital prefer to work in
committees, believing that a collective decision is liable to be
more sound than one made by a single person. Mark counters that
a good head of department would only make decisions after wide
consultation with his or her colleagues.

Catherine is torn between the need for modern efficiencies
and offending her beloved Ethiopians. If the trustees end up being
divided about any decision, Catherine, as the founder, has the last
word. She is not convinced that they have to remain the world
leaders in fistula surgery. 'I don't mind about being the centre
of excellence for fistulas. I don't mind if we're not even known.
If somebody gets ahead of us it doesn't matter to me, as long as
we're helping these women.'

Catherine has never had any doubts about her priorities. The
patients come first. And she's intensely loyal to the Ethiopian

doctors, whom she thinks of as part of her family. She's had a hand in training every one of them. She knows their wives, husbands and children. If they have personal problems, often it's Catherine to whom they turn. She's aware that in Ethiopia, as with everywhere in the world, the cost of living is going up.

'We must keep our doctors happy,' she says. 'But we can't just give the doctors a pay increase without doing [something for] the poor nurses. They're really on pittances. The matron gets about 3000 birr a month, something like that. Not very much. And all the poor men that work in the gardens, and the guards and the rubbish collectors – they have to be all given a bit more.'

I don't envy Catherine having to guide the way into the future. The little hospital that she and Reg nursed into life is growing up fast. Managing it through the next stage of development is going to need wisdom and strength. Catherine's wisdom is undoubted; it's her stamina that I worry about.

CHAPTER 13

Dr Mulu Muleta, the medical director, is one of the most serious people I've ever met. I couldn't imagine her ever telling a joke. She has a perpetually worried look, as if she is weighed down by matters of life and death – which she is. As well as her own patients, she is ultimately responsible for the medical outcomes of up to 3000 women who have surgery each year.

Mulu was the first Ethiopian surgeon to join the staff permanently, back in 1990. Earlier, she'd done a two-month attachment for her postgraduate studies in O&G. At that time all of the surgery – about 500 to 600 procedures a year – was being done by Reg, Catherine and Mamitu, with occasional help from trainees and visiting doctors from overseas. The Hamlins had offered jobs to several senior Ethiopian gynaecologists, but none had been interested in what they perceived as a career backwater. Mulu saw things differently.

'Reg was so nice,' she says. 'Working with them as a couple is something which will shape you; the commitment and the compassion they have for the fistula patients. They are with the patients until they solve each and every part of their problem – not taking just fistula as the problem. They take patients as a whole; they know each patient's history, what's happened to them socially and physically, and they're trying to solve each and every problem.

'Seeing fistula patients coming in depressed, their clothes soaked with urine and faecal material, transforming them and seeing them going home with big smiles – sometimes they can't even believe they are continent – I thought nothing would satisfy me more. That's why I decided to be a fistula surgeon.'

In a corner of Mulu's office there are a couple of lounges beside a low coffee table where the doctors often share their lunchtime *injera*. Mulu is there, and Biruk, who has just returned from addressing a conference in Portugal. Haile and Habte are there too, tearing off bits of *injera* and using it to scoop up the *wat* which is made from the same *shiro* paste (ground chickpeas mixed with spices) that the patients eat. I'd like to have seen Dr Ambaye, who some say is the best fistula surgeon in the world, again but she's spending a year in Britain studying for a masters degree in public health.

It's a good chance to ask the doctors why they choose this specialty when most of their colleagues prefer other aspects of women's medicine. Biruk was teaching at Gonder University in the north-west before he came to Addis to do postgraduate studies, including two months at the Fistula Hospital. 'I was very much impressed by the love Dr Hamlin gave to these women and the care she's still giving to them. When she invited me to join the hospital there was a reluctance of course, but all of that came into my mind. I thought of all the care she was giving and all the satisfaction that I could have. She gave her life to these women, so I decided to be part of it.'

Biruk was worried that he might regret giving up a satisfy-ing teaching career. But the biggest negative for him has turned out to be stress. 'You see pretty young people who are leaking urine continuously, and that really breaks your heart. The other thing is the success itself. Okay, you can fix 90 to 95 per cent of fistulas, but that doesn't necessarily mean the problem ends. There are a lot of other problems that can happen. The patient might not be completely dry, that's one problem; her private organs are destroyed, so her future fertility is at stake; there's a lot of morbidity attached to the injury, so you know even if you close the hole, there are a lot of other problems going to happen to her. That really makes you feel guilty sometimes, because you think, I haven't done my job as an obstetrician/gynaecologist, I haven't cared for my woman.

'The other part is the operation itself. It's a stressful operation. It takes time, there is often a lot of scarring, it's a kind of plastic surgery, so all this makes it very stressful professionally.'

I suggest that most surgeons just do their job and don't get involved.

'I've been operating on other cases and normally that's what I do. I operate, there are not many complications and, also, you probably operate on older patients, so if you remove the uterus or the cervix, so what? She's at the end of her reproductive life, so it doesn't matter that much. But here they are very young women with maybe two-thirds of their life ahead of them, so as a human being you cannot help worrying about the outcome.'

I tell him he's just presented a very good argument for *not* being a fistula surgeon.

He laughs. 'There is the other part, the rewarding part. At least you cure a significant portion of these women and that means a lot, because you give them life. You are restoring them back to society. This part is very rewarding, but definitely there is the other part, which is the stress. I want to emphasise that and tell you fistula work is the kind of work that you should give your life to.'

★

Dr Hailegiorgis Aytenfisu – Haile, to his friends and colleagues – has a roly-poly body and a round, friendly face. He's been here for eight years. Early in his career he spent five years in the country. One hospital he worked in was near the Sudanese border, where the temperature rose to 45 degrees in summer. He practised as a general surgeon and learnt a lot about tropical diseases. He came to Addis for postgraduate studies and he, too, was recruited during his attachment to the hospital. 'One reason I liked working at the Fistula Hospital was that in the OR [operating room] when I held out my hand for an instrument I knew that it would be there. In the government hospital, half the time they have to go and look for it and then you can't be sure that it's been sterilised properly.'

Haile reckons he'll probably be here for life. He doesn't care about giving up lucrative private practice. 'When they get cured, that's the best reward.'

Dr Habtemariam Tekle – Habte – is tall and lean and rather shy. He considers all questions carefully and answers in great detail – a methodical approach that must inspire confidence in his patients. In the early part of his career he also spent time in a rural hospital near the Sudanese border. It had been destroyed during the war with Eritrea and been rebuilt with sticks and mud. Ethiopia was going through a turbulent time. The communist regime which had deposed the former emperor Haile Selassie was about to topple. Many senior staff had fled and Habte was left to cope with everything, from malaria epidemics to amputations. He often couldn't refer serious cases to the big regional hospital at Gonder, as there was only one car in the district, and it could only move in the dry season. So he had to deal with them himself. 'That was a challenge for me at the beginning of my career.'

After two and a half years Habte moved to Gonder, where he

occasionally assisted one of the gynaecologists with simple fistula surgery. He had some more exposure during postgraduate studies in Addis in O&G. When he returned to Gonder, Ambaye and Haile visited on an outreach trip and he assisted them. The siren song of fistula surgery was becoming hard to resist. His fate was sealed when the hospital gave him some equipment and he began doing straightforward cases himself. He came to Addis about a year ago and since then he's been benefiting greatly from working with the experts. 'Cases that seemed difficult in Gonder seem simple to me now. If I have difficult cases I can call for assistance from the others.'

Dr Yifru Terefe Teshome – Yifru – wanted to be a doctor from when he was a small boy growing up in Addis Ababa. After he graduated from high school with top marks, he did his medical training in Addis and was then sent to a small hospital, again near the Sudanese border, to do his compulsory rural service.

They called it a hospital, he says, but it wasn't really. Yifru was the only doctor there. At the end of most days, having dealt with every medical problem imaginable, he was stressed and exhausted. The patients who distressed him most were women in childbirth. He saw women having obstructed labours, or with ruptured uteruses, women near death, and there was very little he could do to help them. Without any surgical instruments, he had to refer them to the nearest properly equipped hospital 300 kilometres away. It was difficult to find transport and the roads were often impassable.

This experience made him decide to study obstetrics and gynaecology. When he did his attachment at the Fistula Hospital he was so impressed with what he saw that he asked for a job there.

Yifru became a doctor because he wanted to help people.

Money is not his first priority. 'I am using my skills to help those who need it, and that satisfies me.'

The second longest serving doctor, after Dr Mulu, is Dr Ambaye Wolde Michael. She, too, heard the call of fistula surgery while on attachment to the hospital during her postgraduate studies. Impressed both by her surgical skill and her heartfelt concern for the patients, Reg invited her to join the staff after she had graduated. The Ministry of Health refused permission, as they wanted her to go elsewhere. Ambaye joined anyway. It was several months before the ministry tracked her down. After some spirited argument from Reg, the bureaucrats relented and allowed her to stay.

Once, when Ambaye was attending a conference in America, some gynaecologists tried to persuade her to live there, telling her she would make a lot of money. She would not be tempted. She loved her country too much, and the needy women she was helping.

It was Ambaye who began the hospital's outreach program, involving trips to distant provincial hospitals to operate. Usually two nurses would go with her – a trained nurse and one of the theatre-trained nurse aides. The hospital Land Rover would be loaded with all the equipment they needed, such as surgical instruments, operating clothes, gloves, catheters, spinal anaesthetics, even gauze and cotton wool. The local hospital would already have collected patients needing surgery and the team would use its operating theatre. Perhaps ten or fifteen women might be waiting when they arrived. Ambaye and the others would also train the hospital staff and do some teaching in the villages about harmful traditional practices, such as early marriage, that contribute to fistula injuries. During her visits to outlying villages Ambaye sometimes discovered victims hidden away from the rest of the world. Many of them were in the most appalling condition after years of suffering. Some owed Ambaye their lives after she had taken them back to Addis to treat their injuries.

When I was here last, Ambaye was living in a house within the hospital compound. She was a keen gardener and also raised chickens, which supplied the hospital with all of its eggs. Since then a few things have changed. In 2001 Ambaye married and moved into a house in town with her husband; the place where the chickens used to roost is now the Oprah Winfrey Centre.

There is great esprit de corps amongst the staff. One day in the Bete Mesgana about 25 people gather for a celebration for Dr Biruk and Tenegne, the woman who runs the lab. Biruk has just earned his masters degree in public health, after two years of study. Tenegne is leaving to go to America for two years' further study. She has been with the hospital since it opened in 1975.

All the doctors are there, plus Matron, some nurses, a few nurse aides and, of course, Catherine and Ruth. On a table in the middle of the room are a large tray of popcorn, warm bottles of Coca-Cola and two big round loaves of bread, one wrapped in white paper and one in pink. Off to one side some nurse aides are preparing the inevitable trays of strong black coffee.

There's lots of joking and giggling as people find their seats. I'm reminded of a rowdy class in school. Dr Haile is the MC. He begins with prayers, then jokingly wonders who should cut which loaf. Someone shouts out, 'Pink for Biruk', and everyone laughs.

Haile makes a gracious speech about the skills of his colleague, Biruk, and how deserving he is; about how much Tenegne will be missed. Then Biruk gets up and speaks. He especially thanks

Catherine – Dr Hamlin – for helping him financially in his studies, and his colleagues for their support.

Tenegne speaks and gets a little teary. Then Catherine gets up and gives them both presents – a gold necklace with a cross for Biruk, a bracelet for Tenegne. Everyone applauds. Biruk and Tenegne smile from ear to ear. Amid laughter, they each cut their loaf of bread. The nurse aides hand round the slices, with coffee, and everyone leaves their seats to come up and congratulate the pair.

These dedicated Ethiopian doctors have worked hard and made many sacrifices to get where they are. They become very prickly when foreign doctors waltz in and do a couple of weeks' training in fistula surgery then go back to their own affluent countries. 'Fistula tourists', they call them. They wouldn't mind if they were going to use their skills in the developing world.

Says Biruk, 'There are people who just want to come here and have some training; some of them don't even bother much about the training, they just want to have some kind of certificate and then they go back and put it on their CV, and probably they'll some day be an authority on fistula.'

The hospital used to be happy to help anyone, but lately they've become much more hard-nosed about who they'll teach. What particularly irks the Ethiopian doctors is the assumption that fistula surgery is easy. Mulu has seen it many times. 'I had senior gynaecologists from America who came to visit once. I assisted one who was the president of the American Gynecological Society. I gave him the chance to do a very small fistula. He couldn't believe it. He said to his friends, "Oh, guys, this is not as simple as it looks. I thought it was easy, watching the experts, but it's not."'

The eight Ethiopian doctors, including Mamitu, plus the three

Europeans, together represent a rich repository of expertise. If Mark Bennett's predictions are correct and the hospital has to compete with other institutions for funding in the future, they have an enviable head start on the rest. The Addis Ababa Fistula Hospital is the standard by which all others are judged.

CHAPTER 14

One visitor the hospital absolutely could not do without is Professor Gordon Williams, the English urologist who's been coming to Ethiopia for twenty years to do the ileal conduit operations. Gordon is a 62-year-old dynamo. We're sitting in Catherine's drawing room one morning when he arrives, fresh off the all-night flight from London. He's smartly dressed, in perfectly pressed brown slacks, a burnt-orange shirt and checked sports jacket, with a natty tie cinched up tight. He's slightly portly, practically bald, his eyes surrounded by laugh lines. He seems always to have a half-smile on his face even when he's serious.

As ever, he comes bearing gifts – Prince Charles biscuits and chocolates for Catherine, a bag full of second-hand trainers and pantyhose for the physiotherapy patients. The trainers are for the women with dropped foot, as they need a big shoe. They cut off the legs of the pantyhose and wear the top part, padded with cloth while they do their exercises. These gifts are collected by students from the Lady Eleanor Holles School at Hampton, west London. They also at Christmas send a card and a bar of scented soap to every patient and staff member. Gordon visits the school regularly to tell them how the hospital is getting on.

Gordon is forceful, sardonic, confident, opinionated, with a ferocious intellect, quoting effortlessly and in detail statistics from clinical studies and surveys. He doesn't hold back on criticism if he thinks things aren't up to standard. He pioneered the kidney transplant scheme at Hammersmith Hospital in London and for the last four years he's been responsible for all the surgical training in Britain. In between teaching and running a busy clinical practice, he finds the time to come to Ethiopia twice a year to operate. In an emergency he's been known to catch the Friday-night flight from London, operate on Saturday and take the next flight home in time to go to work on Monday morning. He never goes on holiday. Quote: 'Three days sitting in the sun is enough for me, then I get bored stiff.'

Gordon first came to Ethiopia as an external examiner for final-year medical students. He'd read the Hamlins' work in the *British Medical Journal*, so decided to look them up. Reg was a great raconteur and Gordon tells a pretty good story himself. Although they weren't urologists, the Hamlins were doing an operation on the bladder, so the three had plenty in common to discuss. Every time he came back he'd call in at the hospital, they'd have lunch and talk about the latest developments in urology. They steered clear of religion, though, as Gordon doesn't believe in God.

'Catherine and I try not to talk about it. I can't imagine how there can be God with so much poverty around. Catherine tells me it's because the Devil influences things. That's put the kybosh on any long-term plans to work here. Not that I worry. I'd get bored stiff doing fistulas all the time.'

The first of many lives that Gordon saved in Ethiopia was that of Letekidane Gebre Yohannes. As related in *The Hospital by the River*, Lete had arrived from northern Shoa province with a dead baby inside her and a history of being in labour for five days. A craniotomy, or compressing of the baby's head, was done and the decomposing baby delivered. Lete's injuries were severe; most of her bladder had been destroyed and what was left had been reduced to the size of a thimble. She underwent many repair operations but was never cured of her urinary incontinence.

Lete was in charge of the hospital outpatients department and one of the stores. She did her work with a ureteric catheter in one of the strictured ureters, draining into a test tube strapped to her leg, or an empty drip-set bag. Gradually her kidneys had become diseased and her life was threatened. The Hamlins had asked a number of visiting surgeons if they could do something, but all refused to operate, predicting that her kidneys would fail if she had further surgery. When they asked Gordon Williams for help he took a more positive view.

'My attitude was if you don't do something she *will* die; if you do, she might not. They didn't do abdominal surgery then, so I brought some equipment from the UK and it took me an hour and a half to sort Lete out. It was absolutely straightforward. The ureters coming from the kidneys to the bladder weren't in her bladder, which had been destroyed. They were stuffed into the side wall of the pelvis. She was getting infections more and more and her kidney function was deteriorating, they were getting wrecked. I did the operation and she lived for another eighteen years as a really useful member of staff here.'

I remembered Lete from my last visit as a small figure limping due to a congenital partial dislocation of the hip. She used to go about her tasks with a solemn expression, obviously loving her job. She shared a *tukul* with Mamitu and another nurse aide, Likelesh.

In 2005 Lete's kidneys began finally to fail. It took her six weeks to die, and it was horrible for her friends to stand by and watch her slowly slipping away. After she had passed away there was deep, deep mourning at the hospital. Lete was in her mid-fifties.

★

On this trip Gordon has five patients to see, all of whom are experiencing complications, such as kidney infections, following ileal conduit operations. They've been discovering these complications only lately, after long-term followup. Gordon thinks it's because of the unique nature of injuries in Ethiopia. 'I think here the conduit is a bit of a problem in that the lower ends of the ureters don't have much blood supply to them. Whereas if you're doing a conduit in the west, it's usually because someone's had their bladder removed due to cancer, and there's no problem with the blood supply. I'm seeing now with increased followup a small number of patients who are developing strictures at the lower end of the conduit.'

The ureters are narrow little tubes, whilst the ileum is relatively wide. They've now changed the operation slightly so that the two ureters are brought together into one before being attached to the ileum. They're re-doing some old operations. 'It's disappointing to come out and see these girls. It's relatively simple to re-implant the ureters, but it's a great shame for the patient to have to undergo another operation.'

And if they didn't do it? The answer is very simple. The patient would die.

Gordon has taught doctors Mulu, Ambaye, Biruk and Haile how to do ileal conduits. There are some cases they could do by themselves, but for the time being they're reluctant to go ahead without him there to guide them. You have to be doing this procedure on a regular basis to learn all the nuances.

Gordon has been twice married and has two daughters, who've given him four grandchildren. He cheerfully acknowledges that his work ethic has had a lot to do with the failures of his marriages. Now he's got a new project, one that is quite breath-

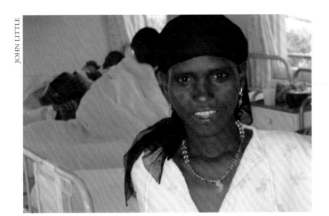

Amina.

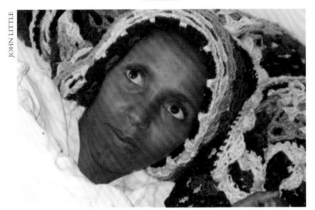

Zemebech.

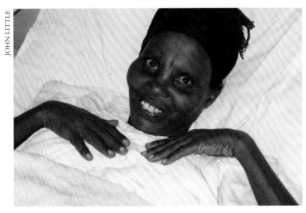

Halema.

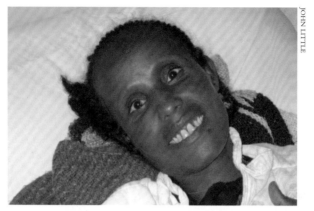

JOHN LITTLE

Alganish.

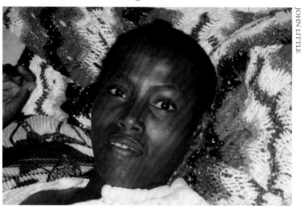

JOHN LITTLE

Leteabazgi.

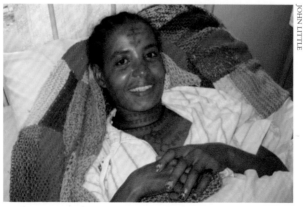

JOHN LITTLE

Letelibanes.

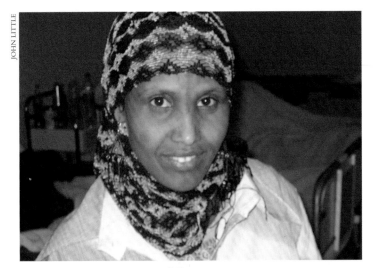

Minsera.

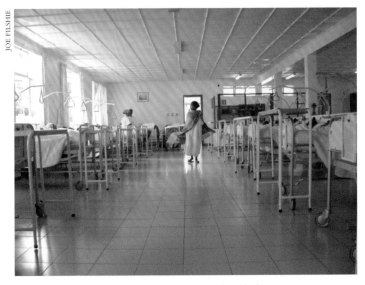

The main ward in Addis Ababa.

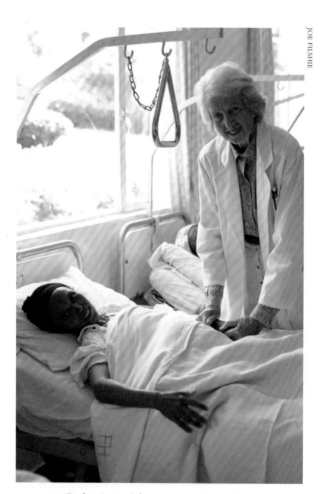

Catherine with a recovering patient.

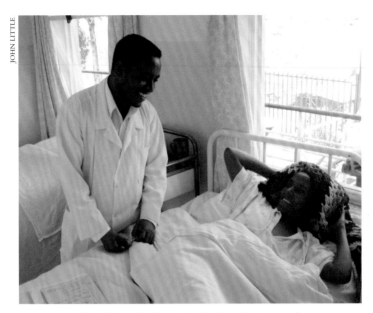

JOHN LITTLE

Dr Abiy tells Zemebech that she is cured.

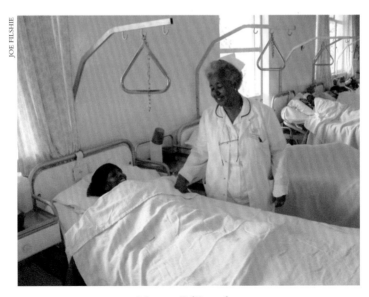

JOE FILSHIE

Matron Edjigayehu.

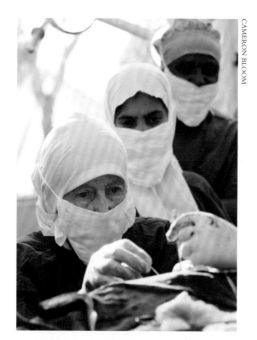

Catherine in the operating room.

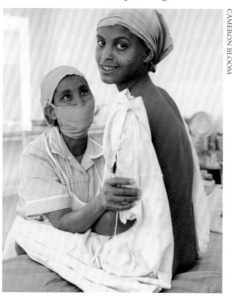

A patient about to receive a spinal
anaesthetic prior to surgery.

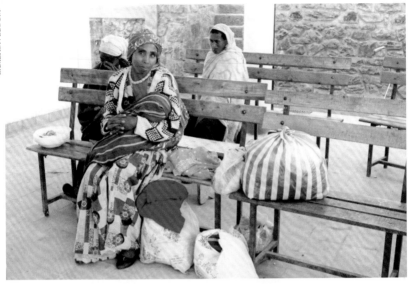

CAMERON BLOOM

New patients wait to be admitted to hospital.

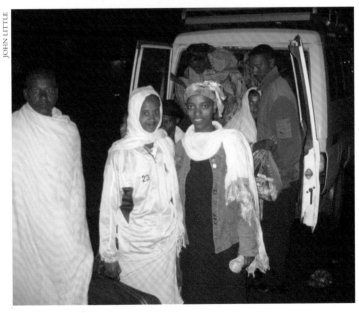

JOHN LITTLE

Cured patients catching the bus to go home.

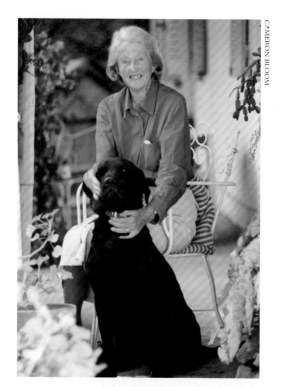

CAMERON BLOOM

Catherine with her faithful Labrador, Chips.

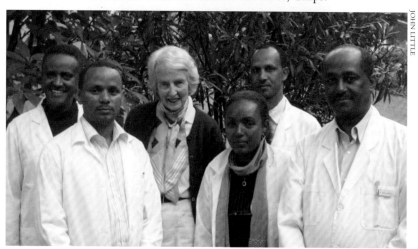

JOHN LITTLE

(Left to right) Dr Biruk, Dr Yifru, Dr Hamlin, Dr Mulu, Dr Habte and
Dr Haile.

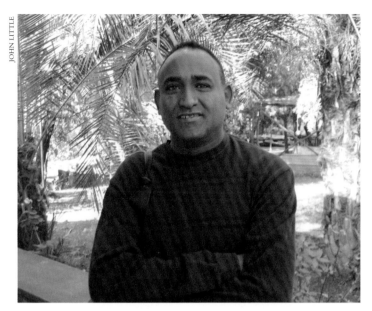

Dr Melaku, in charge of the Mekele hospital.

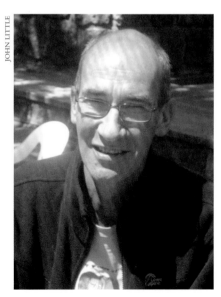

Dr Einar, in charge of Yirgalem.

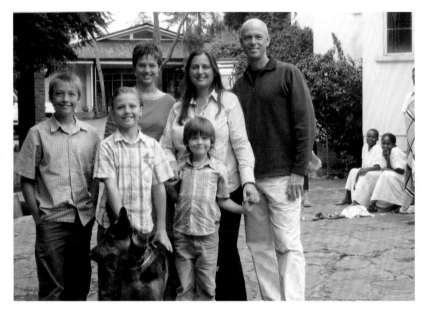

Mark and Annette Bennett with their daughter, Alleysia, and
sons (left to right) Lewis, Martin and Dylan.

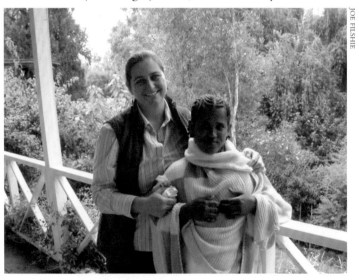

Annette Bennett with a young patient.

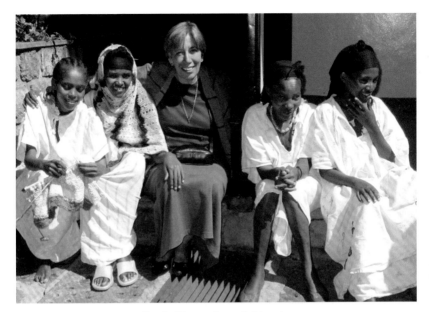

Ruth Kennedy and friends.

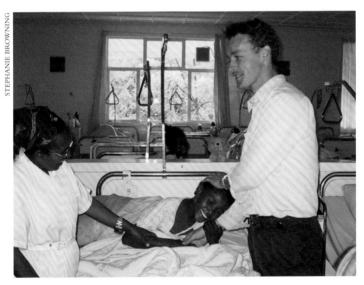

STEPHANIE BROWNING

Andrew Browning with a very happy patient.

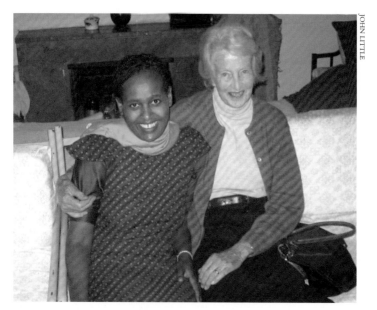

Catherine and Wokinesh.

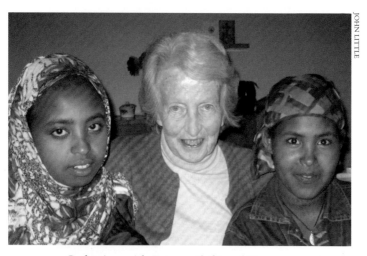

Catherine with Fatuma (left) and Bossena.

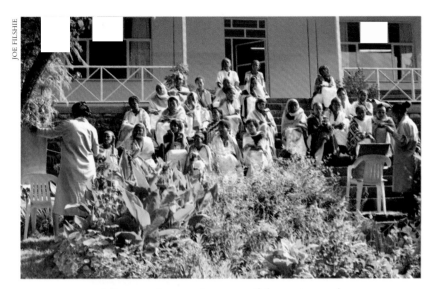

A literacy class on the steps of the main ward.

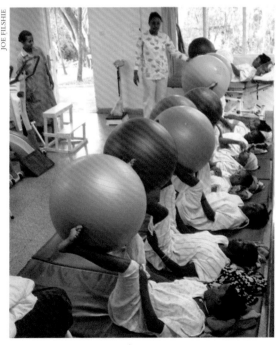

A physiotherapy session at Addis Ababa.

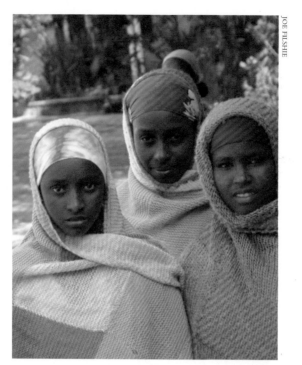

JOE FILSHIE

Recovering patients wearing shawls donated to
the hospital.

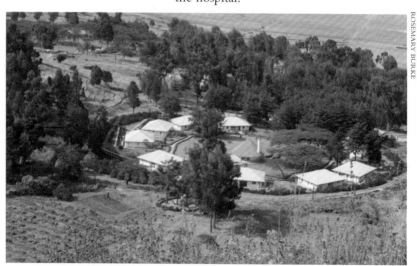

ROSEMARY BURKE

Desta Mender (Joy Village), home for incurable patients.

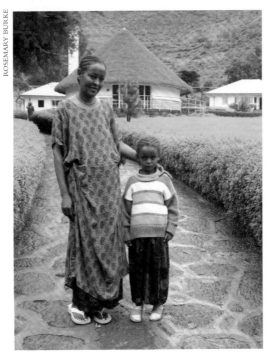

Louise Nicholson reunited with some old friends.

Habite and her daughter, Rachel, at Desta Mender.

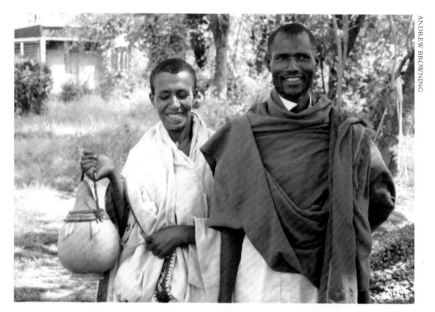

A cured patient returns to Bahar Dar with a present of milk.

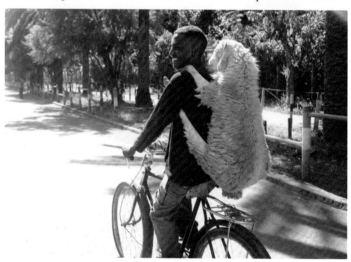

The Brownings' meat supply arrives.

taking in its ambition. He wants to found a medical school with a radical curriculum specially tailored for a developing country.

There's a critical shortage of doctors in the rural areas. Gordon cites a review of Gonder Hospital which illustrates the point. It is the only hospital for 21 million people. For a year there was no patient in the surgical wards who lived more than 100 kilometres from Gonder. The conclusion was that if you lived more than a 100 kilometres away with a life-threatening condition, you'd die.

He points out that at present the top 500 graduates in the national school exam are told they have to do medicine whether they want to be doctors or not. Lots of them don't have any particular desire to serve humanity, and as soon as they can after graduation, they're on the plane to America or Saudi Arabia, where the big money is.

Thirty per cent of the students at Gordon's school will come from poorer parts of Ethiopia. They won't have to be at the top academically. They'll complete a formal application form, get a reference from the principal and go before an interviewing committee, including a woman and a medical student from an adjacent medical school who will be recognised by his or her peers as being 'the right sort of person for sorting out who's likely to make a good doctor'.

Gordon's syllabus will be more basic than the standard one. 'What they have now is a masters degree in medicine, which is seven years. It's a complete waste of time. They don't need to know as much as they're being taught. They need a bachelors degree, which is five years; I want them to do a two-year program with periods of four months – four months in the community, four in obstetrics, four in surgery, four in acute medicine, four in paediatrics and perhaps four in psychiatry. So when they leave they can do simple procedures such as strangulated hernias or an appendix.

'After three or four years if they're really making a difference in the rural area, some can come back and undergo further training and become a specialist. So there is a pathway for them. If they work hard and show they're continuing to learn, we can bring them back and they can become a cardiologist or a paediatrician or whatever.'

Gordon speaks as if he has no doubts that his school will happen. But there are enormous obstacles to overcome – money is one, and perhaps the most formidable of them is the Ethiopian bureaucracy. He's got appointments with the Health Department, the Education Department and a university where he wants his school to be.

Catherine and Ruth are listening to his plans with a sort of amused tolerance. More than anyone, they know what he's up against. There's no stopping him, though. He tells them that he's just spent a million birr, which he raised in England through charitable contributions, on equipment for his as yet non-existent school. But the bureaucrats don't seem to be quite as driven as he is. For instance, he thinks they should be taking advantage of the millennium, which under the Ethiopian calendar falls this year. 'You've got the diaspora coming in their thousands. What are they doing to tap them? Nothing. What are they doing to show them how inadequate the hospitals are so they might donate some money? Nothing. I'm in constant e-mail communication with them. I'm going mad.'

'Don't go mad yet,' says Catherine.

A couple of days later I catch up with Gordon to see how he's getting on. He seems to have lost a bit of his fizz. He went to the Ministry of Education for a long-scheduled meeting which was due to last all day, and no one knew anything about it.

A few days after that, Ruth and I have dinner with him at an

Italian restaurant. The owner, a big fleshy man with an exaggerated Italian accent, and the flamboyant gestures to match, greets him effusively. Gordon likes his food, and he's a regular here every time he visits. The illusion of Italy is carried through inside. There are white tablecloths, and waiters with white aprons, although when they speak, the accent is Ethiopian not Italian. The clientele all seems to be European. I cannot see one Ethiopian.

Gordon scans the menu, which features proper Italian cuisine, and the list of imported wines; he orders lamb and chips. The chips here are first rate, he tells us. We really should try them.

He's still having problems with the bureaucracy. The administration wants him to be attached to St Paul's University but he can't find the chancellor, who hasn't got a mobile phone. The five medical schools in the country are run by the Ministry of Education. The Ministry of Health runs hospitals. They're fed up with the outcomes, so he's setting up his school under the Ministry of Health. He's now discovered that the curriculum he wants has to go to a national curriculum committee, run by – you guessed it, the Ministry of Education. It's the usual bureaucratic roundabout. He's worried, because when he's heard his Ethiopian coordinating doctor talk to the minister, a lot of what he's saying just isn't right. Sometimes he feels like saying, 'That's not true at all, we're not doing that.'

He has to decide in the next ten days whether to resign all his posts in Britain and come to live in Ethiopia. He's due to fly home at midnight tomorrow and nothing has been resolved. He seems a little glum, but after an intake of chips and a passable red he's upbeat again, talking about finding a place to live and whether or not to bring his furniture out. 'It's time for a new challenge,' he enthuses. 'What the hell, I might as well give it a go.'

The following evening Gordon comes to the hospital to say goodbye. We're sitting in Catherine's drawing room when he suddenly turns pale and sways on his feet. He clutches at Catherine's desk and lowers himself into a chair; he's breathing heavily and his face is wet with perspiration. He's a little over-weight. That and the stress he's under . . . well, it makes you think. It's a quarter of an hour before he recovers enough to walk up the path to the car waiting to take him to the airport. Despite all of his difficulties, his enthusiasm for the school remains undiminished.

When we've said our goodbyes I ask Catherine if she thinks he'll succeed. 'I think he might have trouble,' she says. 'He's really impatient. It's amazing that he's suddenly wanted to do it. He said to me once, "You've made an enormous difference to my life." I said, "Gordon, why?" He said, "I've got a new lease of life by coming here."'

What he's doing seems completely impractical for someone at his stage of life but there's something about this hospital, and its founder, which inspires people to look beyond safety and comfort. From the most humble medical student to an acclaimed professor, no one is immune.

The great drawback to the ileal conduit operation is that the women can no longer live in their village without medical help at hand. The Fistula Hospital is the only place in Ethiopia importing the stoma bags. In many other developing countries they are simply not an option. Some years ago well-meaning French surgeons did ileal conduit operations on two women in Chad. It was only after they had done the procedure, bringing the ureters out to the stomach wall, that they discovered stoma bags were not available. Life for those two women had not changed. The only difference was that they were leaking from a different place.

There are alternative diversion operations, where the urine drains through the anus. One method is to put the ureters directly into the sigmoid colon, the last part of the large bowel. The drawback is that you get faecal matter going back up to the kidneys and lots of infections. And it sometimes leads to cancer later.

That operation has been pretty well abandoned now. A better procedure is to fold the sigmoid together, cut along it and make it into a pouch. The ureters are put into that pouch and the urine eventually drains into the main part of the colon, where it mixes with faecal matter. Advocates of the operation say that there's very little infection. It can lead to some electrolytic abnormality, but that can easily be fixed by taking sodium bicarbonate, which can be bought in any small town.

The operation is called the Mainz II pouch, after the town in Germany where it was developed. Gordon, for one, is all for it, and can't understand why his colleagues in Addis Ababa aren't quite so enthusiastic. 'They should be doing it with lots of these girls who have conduit and infection problems, but they're not doing it. It's stupid. They're continent, they don't need a bag and they can go home and live a normal life, but they won't do it.

'When I come here permanently I'm going to say I'm not going to do any more conduits unless the anal sphincter is not intact. Get a bag of saline or water and put a little tube into the anus, inject three or four hundred cc, get the girl to walk around and if she can hold that, then she can have a pouch.'

Catherine has reservations about abandoning ileal conduits. 'The bag is still the best solution,' she says. 'With the pouch, urine and faeces can still mix together. There is still a risk of infection. If a woman has only one kidney or has compromised kidney function this can be dangerous.'

The medical director, Dr Mulu, is also urging a cautious approach. The operation is only about twelve years old. She thinks that more time is needed to see what the long-term outcomes will be.

CHAPTER 15

The outreach hospital at Bahar Dar is a plain, rectangular building in a field off to one side of the government hospital. It looks more like a warehouse or a factory than a hospital. There's none of the landscaping or lovingly cultivated flower beds which distinguish the complex at Addis Ababa. Only the presence of a few women in hospital gowns, sitting outside the front entrance, and a smattering of ragged new arrivals, indicate its purpose. The front entrance gives onto a hallway, on one side of which is an examination room. On the other side is a reception area and a teaching room where patients can learn basic reading and writing and learn about the story of Jesus if they wish. Beyond is the main ward with 45 beds. It's laid out in similar fashion to Addis, with four rows of beds divided down the middle by a low wall. At the far end a door opens onto the doctors' changing-room and the operating theatre.

There are two tables in the theatre. Andrew Browning, dressed in the usual green scrubs, is working at one when I arrive. He has a caver's light on his head, in case one of the regular black-outs occurs. Bahar Dar is what Addis must have been like in the early days. They've had two periods of ten days when they had no water. They were collecting water from the drainpipes off the roof. A few days ago there was a monkey looking through the window of the OR.

A young Ugandan obstetrician, Dr Mwange Moses, is at the other table. Dr Mwange is here for a month to learn about fistula surgery. Andrew has a reputation as a first-class teacher. Foreign students often ask for him specifically when they come to study.

Andrew is a man in a hurry. He speaks so rapidly that sometimes his tongue can't keep up with the words. Consequently he's a little hard to understand at times, especially when he's using medical terms. At Bahar Dar he does about 650 operations a year, which is more than in Addis. Everything happens faster at Bahar Dar. He has refined his technique by doing, for example, fewer sutures, so that his operations take less time. Instead of recuperating in bed for a fortnight, his patients are up and walking on day one. They wander about holding little plastic buckets, into which their catheters drain. These innovations have not compromised the outcomes. In fact, they're as good as or better than in Addis.

When Andrew's not operating, examining new patients, doing rounds or attending to administration, he's doing research, writing papers, attending conferences, and pondering new ways to solve the last great challenge of fistula surgery: stress incontinence. He's invented a new operation which, in the short term at least, has considerably reduced its incidence in his patients.

In his own country, Australia, he could have had a brilliant, well-paid career. He came from a Christian family. His father was an obstetrician/gynaecologist, and from the time he was a little boy Andrew wanted to be a missionary doctor. When he was a medical student he did an elective in Tanzania. It was the beginning of the Rwanda crisis and he saw hundreds of dead bodies floating down the rivers. Working in hospitals and refugee camps with victims of the atrocities, he decided that this was what he wanted to do with his life.

Back in Australia he did a couple of years of junior medicine at Gosford near Sydney. He then had a stint with his aunt, Valerie Browning, a nurse working with the Afar nomads in the desert of northern Ethiopia. He wanted to see if he'd like to go there permanently. The Afar region is one of the hottest and poorest places on earth. It was about 35 degrees in winter while he was there. At the end of one long day doing a clinic in the middle of nowhere, he and his health workers killed a sheep and ate dinner. Then, complaining of the cold, his companions retired to a hut with an open fireplace. It was miserably hot, so Andrew went outside to sleep. An armed guard had to bunk down beside him to ward off hyenas. Every time Andrew started to drop off, the guard would fire a couple of shots and wake him up. The hyenas eventually got the message, but his sleep was interrupted yet again by a cow giving birth a few metres away. The calf flopped out onto the ground and Andrew was splashed with amniotic fluid. He began to think that working under these conditions might not be for him.

His father had told him about the Fistula Hospital. He started dropping in whenever he was in Addis. Catherine would give him lunch and invite him into the theatre, where he assisted her a few times. Catherine must have sensed the passion waiting to burst into life because she ended up suggesting that he might like to come and work there one day.

Andrew went back home to do a year of theology training. During that time he thought about her offer, prayed about it and came to the same conclusion as others who've fallen under the spell of fistula surgery. As he puts it, 'There are so few operations you can do that can transform someone's life.'

He knew that if he really wanted to be a fistula surgeon he'd have to study O&G. While he was doing his postgraduate course he made more short trips to Ethiopia. Catherine, Ambaye, Mulu and Mamitu were the only ones doing surgery then. 'It was

Mamitu,' he says, 'who taught me everything I know.'

In the theatre Mwange is having trouble. He calls Andrew over. He peers at the operation site for a few moments then guides Mwange through some intricate suturing at a spot so far inside the body that he's working as much by touch as by sight. After a few minutes Mwange's looking a lot more confident. During his month here he will do 20 to 25 operations of increasing difficulty. It takes a lot more than 25 to become an accomplished fistula surgeon. Today Andrew saw Mwange's limit. He's got another difficult one for him in a couple of days' time.

Andrew's last patient is a girl who looks about twelve years old. Her eyes are wide with fright. Andrew gives her the spinal himself, as they have no anaesthetist. She has a small fistula which Andrew closes in twenty minutes. He's confident that she'll be cured.

The two surgeons take off their scrubs, Andrew writes up his notes and it's time for the ward round. The patients are all waiting with their little buckets under their beds. The tubes cost a couple of cents in the hardware store and the buckets cost about a dollar and last a year, so they're a lot cheaper than urine bags, which cost about ten dollars and only last for one person.

The first patient is called Emway. She can't stop smiling. 'If they're dry when they're walking around,' says Andrew, 'it's a good indication that they're not going to be incontinent.' Emway is showing all the right indicators, so they can pretty well guarantee that she's going to be cured.

By contrast, the patient in the next bed looks very sorry for herself. 'This one's impossible,' says Andrew. 'She was operated on in Addis nineteen years ago. Completely failed. Then she was operated on here in December last year and again failed. Both rectally and vesically [in the bladder]. There's no vagina, just rock-solid scar. So this is the third go. Each time we operate, the chance of succeeding becomes less.'

A nurse lifts the sheet and he examines his unhappy patient. He questions the nurse and shakes his head. The patient is wet.

'Cases like these make you a bit disappointed,' he says. 'You know you're going to put yourself through an awful operation, give yourself and the patient headaches and it's not going to do her much good. Sometimes you're surprised, though. Maybe she'll do okay. You've got to give them the chance, because it's the only chance they've got.'

The next patient is a perfect illustration of why Andrew never likes to give up hope. 'She had an enormous fistula but the urethra was intact, which was the thing that was going for her. Both ureters were stuck in scar. They were tiny little pinholes just squirting a little bit of urine. We cut away that scar and there were big dilated ureters behind. So we relieved that obstruction to the kidney because over time it will destroy the kidneys and she'll die from chronic renal failure. Then we closed the fistula, but in closing the fistula the bladder was tiny, because most of it had been destroyed by the long labour. We were certain that she was going to be a hopeless case, because we couldn't even blow up the balloon of the catheter in the bladder, it was so small. I took the catheter out after one day, as there was no point in leaving it, it was just going to fall out all the time. I left the ureteric catheters in for about twelve days while the implantation into the bladder healed, then took them out, and miraculously she was dry! So the bladder must have stretched pretty quickly, and she was cured.'

The patient in the next bed, Athris, is fifteen. Her first baby was stillborn after three days of labour. Hers was a small fistula which they had repaired yesterday. She's dry, drinking and draining. Unusually, her husband is still around, so her story may turn out to have a happy ending too.

We move on to another positive story – that of a woman with

a baby daughter lying beside her and another daughter, about seven years old, standing by the bed. She's an ex-fistula patient. The seven-year-old was her first child, the second, stillborn, gave her a fistula. When they repaired her they told her that she should have her next child in hospital. She came to them about a week before the baby was due and had a caesarean in the government hospital next door. Andrew says that ex-patients generally take his advice about getting to hospital early. The trouble is they do get some who develop another fistula. Usually it's because she's married another husband who doesn't understand the problem, hasn't seen it for himself and won't let her go to the hospital. The attitude is, my mother delivered in the village without any problems, so why shouldn't you?

The next patient had been carried in on a litter the day before. She can't walk because of contractures. They've started her on physiotherapy. Andrew says they'll get her legs working, then operate.

And so it goes, about twenty patients in all. Most with good outcomes, and a few who just break my heart. We finish the round and go into the outpatients department to see today's new arrivals. The first is a girl called Bosie from South Gonder, about 80 kilometres away. She's dressed in a very dirty *gabi*, wearing a necklace with a big cross; she has tattoos down her jawline. Bosie says she's twenty years old. She arrived yesterday with the patient who was carried in with contractures. It turns out she's Bosie's aunt.

Bosie has had two children, both born dead. With the second one she had a retained placenta, so she went to a health centre. After they removed it she says she developed a fistula. She's been leaking urine for seven years. If that's true I think she must be older than twenty. But they're always a bit vague about their ages.

Bosie is divorced and lives with her mother, who's waiting

outside. Andrew examines her and pronounces that there's a
99 per cent possibility of cure.

I'm curious to hear more about how two women from the
same family ended up with fistulas. Outside, Bosie's mother
sits patiently on a log with her travelling things on the ground
beside her. She has a leather pot in which she carries food, a
plastic water bottle, an umbrella and a couple of plastic bags with
spare clothes. She looks desperately poor. Her *gabi* is grey with
dirt and her hands are callused from work. I'd guess her age at
about 40.

She tells me through a hospital translator that it took a day's
travel on foot then an 80-kilometre bus ride to get here from
her village. Her sister – Bosie's aunt – has been married twice.
She had eight children by her first husband, then he died. She
remarried and became pregnant to her new husband. When
she went into labour the baby's head appeared but no matter how
hard she tried to push it out it would come no further. The traditional birth attendant advised her to go to a health centre, so they
rounded up some people from the village and carried her there
on a litter. The health centre said that the case was beyond them,
so they put her on the litter once more, still with the baby half
born, and carried her to another health centre. There the baby
was stillborn. By then she had been in labour for three days.

When it was noted that she had a fistula, the second health
centre advised her to go to hospital, but the five friends who'd
carried her had to get back for the harvest. There was no way to
get her there without them, so they took her home.

The aunt's husband left her soon afterwards and then she
got sick with fever. The family was reluctant to take her to the
hospital because of what had happened to Bosie, whose injuries,
they believed, had been caused by the people at the health centre.
It was only when one of the aunt's sons, who was a student at
Bahar Dar, came home and insisted that she go, that they made

the journey.

I ask how she thinks her daughter's fistula happened. She says she thinks that someone at the health centre must have poked a hole by accident.

The aunt's father, Bosie's grandfather, wanders over and joins us. He's an old man, his face deeply lined from a lifetime working in the fields. He carries a staff. He's wearing a pair of ragged shorts and has a *gabi* thrown over his shoulder. His horny old feet are bare and caked with mud. The translator explains to them how fistulas are caused. They listen with rapt attention then ask a lot of questions. Bosie's mother is incredulous. She says she's had six children at home without any problem. Now she's worried. Her last child has just got married at the age of twelve. She's not happy living with her husband. She's told her mother she'd rather go to school.

There's a line of women outside outpatients, all with puddles under their feet. In the examination room Andrew sees a former patient who's come in for a six-month followup visit. He goes over her notes. She first had intercourse at the age of seven. The trauma caused a big tear in the rectum. Her husband left her and she lived with the fistula for the next 33 years. Interestingly, she remarried and had three children while she had the fistula. Andrew repaired her and advised her not to have intercourse for six months. Now she's back for her progress to be assessed. She tells Andrew that she's done exactly what he told her to do. He examines her and tells her she's fine. She can start living a normal life again.

The next woman to come into the room looks as though she bears the weight of some great sadness. The corners of her mouth are drawn down and it seems painful for her to walk. She tells Andrew that she's in a lot of pain and is leaking urine all the time.

Andrew can speak basic Amharic but usually gets one of the nurses to translate so there can be no mix-ups. Gradually her story emerges. Three months ago she had an assisted delivery at Gonder Hospital. After a two-day labour the baby was born alive, but it died a day later. She was sent home leaking urine, and told to come back after three months. This is the usual procedure; fistula surgery is difficult soon after birth because the tissues are too fragile. After the three months had passed she came back to Gonder and they referred her here.

Andrew asks her to get onto the table and gets Mwange to do the examination. He takes a look and does a bit of a double take. There's something very puzzling here. He peers more closely and inserts a probe. There seems to be something inside. Andrew goes over and has a look too. They're mystified. Andrew takes a pair of forceps and slowly pulls out a large piece of gauze. The urine has been soaking into it and drying out. The calcium and minerals have been turning the gauze into stone.

The patient gasps with pain as it comes out. The smell is appalling. They dispose of the gauze and examine her once more. High up inside they discover a small fistula.

Andrew surmises that perhaps she was bleeding after the delivery and someone at the hospital decided to pack the vagina, which is not the correct treatment, and then they probably just forgot about her. He shakes his head at such criminal incompetence. 'She's 28 years old, poor thing, she's got no kids and she's been through all this. She could have had toxic shock and died.'

The good thing is she's still married and the fistula is repairable. She has endured this entire distressing ordeal without a word of complaint.

Andrew sees a lot of strange things in outpatients. One of the strangest was when he examined a woman and found what he first thought was a catheter that someone had left inside her. When he looked more closely he saw that in fact it was a large intestinal worm. He surmised that there must be a rectal fistula and it had come from the bowel. Sure enough right up on the cervix there was a little rectal fistula. The worm must have crawled through there and stuck in the vagina.

Andrew lives in Bahar Dar with his wife, Stephanie, and their two-year-old son, William. How they came to be together is a story which you could never write as fiction because the coincidences are too unbelievable. Stephanie spent her first eighteen years in Tanzania, living for some time in the same house where Andrew later lived as a medical student. Her father had worked as a pharmacist in the same hospital in which Andrew worked. He and Stephanie met while Andrew was doing a short attachment with the Flying Doctor Service in Broken Hill. They were attracted to one another, but geography was against them. He soon had to return to Sydney while she stayed behind working as a teacher. Then Stephanie came to Sydney to go to Bible college. They began seeing each other and after a couple of years became engaged. After just two weeks Stephanie broke it off. Andrew was fixated on Africa, while she had grave reservations about returning there. She had enjoyed growing up in Tanzania, but from what she'd heard about Ethiopia she had no illusions about how hard it would be for foreigners to work effectively there.

In 2001 Andrew moved to Ethiopia to work at the hospital permanently. In the meantime Stephanie felt she had been called to be a missionary. She had experienced what she describes as 'a powerful vision' in her church in Sydney, which allayed her fears about Ethiopia. She applied to the Sudan Interior Mission. Of the jobs available the most suitable one for her was at a school in Addis Ababa.

When she moved to Addis, Andrew had been there about

six months. She was staying 2 kilometres up the road from the hospital, the closest they'd ever lived to one another. There was only a small expatriate community in Addis, she was the sole other single Australian in the country, and they'd been engaged before. 'Our arms were twisted,' says Andrew.

It's always fascinating to hear different accounts of the same event. Andrew tends to dwell on the more entertaining aspects of the wedding, of which there were many. On the morning of the big day Stephanie and her bridesmaids, who'd come from Australia, were due to be picked up by a hire car and taken to the hairdresser. The car didn't turn up. Andrew went to the office and found it closed. He rang the owner, who apologised and promised to send a man around.

'When?'

'Oh, about ten o'clock.'

'That's when the wedding's due to start.'

With the car sorted out, Andrew went to pick up the flowers. Stephanie had discussed the arrangements in detail with the florist a week before. When he arrived the florist's staff hadn't even started to prepare them. They bunched a few roses together and tied them up with a bit of string and Andrew went to pick up Stephanie from the hairdresser to get dressed. By then the wedding was due to begin. He was still wearing tracksuit pants and had not yet shaved.

'I quickly had a shave, and threw on my suit, Stephanie came and we had a few happy snaps at the hospital, with all the patients looking on and having a great old time. Then we got married and one of my guests had food poisoning and was vomiting in the garden.'

While Andrew enjoys making a good story out of it, Stephanie has softer memories. Her dress, made of white silk and Italian lace, was beautiful; her veil and tiara, ordered over the internet, were all she had wished for. Catherine decorated the church, while Andrew's aunt, Valerie, and her husband, Ismael, provided an Afar band. Two hundred people assembled in the church and when the service finally happened it was a great success.

The wedding night was spent in five-star luxury at the Sheraton hotel. Then they went to Bahar Dar for the honeymoon, where, notes Andrew: 'We both got dysentery and fleas.'

Bahar Dar is on the shores of Lake Tana, the source of the Blue Nile – or so it is said – the real source is at a spring called Gish Abay, which flows into the lake and out at Bahar Dar where the Blue Nile begins. Bahar Dar is probably as nice a place as you'd find for a honeymoon in Ethiopia. They were only there for two days and were so exhausted that they spent most of the time sleeping.

This very Ethiopian story had a very Ethiopian ending. Andrew and Stephanie were both anxious to get back to Addis to see their friends and families who had come over for the wedding. They hadn't had much chance to talk to them, with all the preparations, and it would probably be years before Andrew and Stephanie saw them again. The couple confirmed their flight back to Addis on Ethiopian Airlines, went out to the airport and were informed that they were not on the passenger list. They were told to stand by in case someone didn't turn up. A few other passengers seemed to be having the same difficulty. They all waited. The aeroplane landed and passengers began to board. No one else had come to the ticket counter. As the last passenger boarded, a limousine drove out onto the tarmac, five VIPs emerged and went up the stairs. When Andrew went to the office to complain he was told, 'No, no, you missed your flight.'

They managed to fly to Addis the next day. After Andrew wrote a letter of complaint, the airline agreed to pay for their extra day's accommodation. At the time of writing he still hadn't cashed the cheque, as it's necessary to spend hours in person at the bank. Time is the one thing he just never seems to have.

In contrast to Andrew's hyperactive disposition, Stephanie is serene, which is just as well, for the life of a *ferenji* in Bahar Dar is not easy. They've had stones thrown at their car a few times, Andrew has had things tossed at him while riding his bike with William, Stephanie has had fruit thrown at her in the market. The natural dislike of foreigners seems to be more acute here than in most places.

They have to tread carefully when it comes to their Christian faith. A couple of years ago an evangelical minister was shot and killed by Orthodox extremists. They can't get *ferengi* food in Bahar Dar. Stephanie buys grain and takes it to a mill to have it ground, then bakes her own bread. Every few weeks they buy a sheep, slaughter it in the back yard and freeze the meat. If they haven't been to Addis for a while they end up living on lamb and carrots and cabbage. The lamb would better be described as mutton – and tough old mutton, at that. The locals don't sell a sheep until it is very old.

Stephanie is unfazed by the hardships. She can see herself spending twenty or 30 years in Africa, although when William gets older and needs to go to school they may have to consider some other place, such as East Africa.

*

Andrew is 37. His passion for surgery has not diminished since he came to Ethiopia six years ago. He's done about 2000 fistula operations. It's a satisfying feeling for him to know that he can handle any case that comes up, no matter how complicated. Every now and then he has to deal with a medical challenge which would stretch the resources of the most well-equipped hospital in the western world. One such was a 40-year-old woman who came to them two weeks after having a caesarean section in one of the government hospitals. She'd endured four days of labour, culminating in a ruptured uterus and a double fistula. The hospital had tried to repair the uterus and then discharged her earlier than they should have. When she came to Bahar Dar she was unconscious, paralysed from the waist down, and blind – corneal ulcers had formed after she'd been lying in a coma at home with her eyes open for about a week. She was riddled with sepsis, her whole body was swollen and she was having trouble breathing.

'We thought she was going to die at any minute,' Andrew recalls. 'Her husband came with her and he had to leave to look after two other kids back home. He said his goodbyes and went away fully expecting never to see his wife again.'

Without the diagnostic tools normally available in a western hospital, much of the treatment plan was formulated by using gut feeling and acumen. The swelling told Andrew that his patient had lost a lot of protein. 'The sepsis probably affected the kidneys, so less protein in the blood means fluids go out through the tissues and your whole body swells up. She was unconscious and we needed to give her drugs and fluids intravenously, but her vascular system was so shut down and she was so swollen we couldn't find a vein. I even cut down onto the veins on her legs without success. We eventually found a vein in her neck, which was a bit difficult as we didn't have any of the longer canulas that you should usually use there. Anyway, it stayed there long enough to treat her.'

With her lungs full of fluid, getting her to breathe properly was urgent. They gave her Lasix, a drug which makes the kidneys force out fluid. It was also critical that they give her oxygen, but there was none available in the whole region, so they had an oxygen concentrator flown up from the Addis hospital. This is a device that sucks the oxygen out of the air and concentrates it. With that they were able to settle her breathing down.

They drained her abdomen of pus and put her on masses of antibiotics. They needed to give her potassium and calcium. The normal procedure is to balance how much fluid is going in with the amount coming out. Because of her fistula there was no way they could gauge the amount of urine that was coming out, so they made an educated guess.

She was completely paralysed from the waist down. 'I've got no idea why,' says Andrew. 'We just gave her physio on her legs; after a while her muscles started to strengthen and she was eventually able to walk.'

They treated her corneal ulcers with Gentamycin and Cholamphenicol and shut her eyes. In time they healed.

She still continued to get fevers, and her uterus was 'full of muck', so they needed to do a curette (a procedure where the walls of the uterus are scraped). 'We don't have curette equipment so we had to go to the government hospital and try to use theirs. It was absolutely rusted and filthy, half the stuff was broken. So we cleaned it up, improvised some Heath Robinson repairs and tried to do our best with it. We did the curette, then drained her abdomen a second time.

'We had to give her blood,' Andrew continues. 'She was dreadfully anaemic and she had no protein. Normally back home in Australia we give them intravenous albumin or Haemaccel to increase the fluid-holding capacity in the blood. The only thing you can get in this region is whole blood. We tried to get whole blood, but there was none, so we had to go to the town, find a couple of boys, screen them for HIV and pay them 100 birr each to give blood.

'There were no blood-giving sets in the region so we had

to get blood-giving sets flown up from Addis. We gave her a couple of pints of blood and at last she started to gain strength, to talk again and breathe properly.'

After about five or six weeks the patient was well enough to be operated on. Both of her fistulas were repaired successfully.

'I don't know how she was cured,' says Andrew. 'I think she was cured miraculously, because I learnt a saying when I was a medical student which is, "God heals and doctors get paid for it." I think this is a case, because we prayed more than we did anything for her.'

The most satisfying moment came when her husband returned two months later expecting to find that his wife had died. He was so overjoyed at her recovery that he went home and brought back a sheep as a present – it was a two-day journey each way.

The people who pass through the doors of this little hospital are the poorest of the poor, yet they find ways to show their gratitude, which makes all the struggle worthwhile. One woman, after being cured, walked six hours to her village then six hours back again to present Andrew with a gourd of milk – a very sour gourd of milk by that time, but a touching gesture nonetheless.

Another of Andrew's patients showed her gratitude by helping a fellow sufferer. She had endured ten months of misery in her village before coming to the hospital. She couldn't even beg because she smelled so bad. She scraped by on food given to her by her family. She had a bladder fistula which was easily cured. When she was able to leave, she went home and started a little business making *injera* and selling it. She found a room to rent and was making a life for herself. Then she discovered another fistula patient who was being neglected just as she had been. She took her into her home and looked after her, and when she had raised enough money for the fares, walked her for six hours to the nearest road, flagged down a truck and travelled three days to Bahar Dar. She stayed with her during her three weeks in hospital, helping with her care, then took her back home. Cured.

Andrew Browning has built up a very successful hospital in Bahar Dar. Through writing papers and speaking at forums he's built an international reputation as an authority on fistula surgery. Yet, fame and fortune do not interest him. 'At the end of the day I'm happy just plodding away here doing my best for the patients.'

CHAPTER 16

Whilst I've been in Bahar Dar I've been wondering how 'my' patients have been getting on back in Addis Ababa. The first thing I do when I return is check up on them. I go looking for Amina. She's not in the main ward where I saw her last. I'm told that she's moved to the Bethlehem ward. I walk in that direction along flagstone pathways bordered by beds of flowers. It's a balmy, sunny morning. About a dozen girls are sitting on the broad steps which run from the main ward down to a sweeping lawn, learning to read and write. The teacher has set up an easel with the Amharic alphabet on it. As she points to each letter, the class says it out loud. It reminds me of my own schooling, back in the days when we used to learn things by rote.

Outside the physiotherapy department Lingersh is at her usual place, holding onto a post doing her leg exercises. Since our interview she no longer looks away when I pass by, but gives me a shy smile. The two men who sweep the paths each morning wish me a cheery good morning in English. One of the nurses walking towards the main ward does the same. I'm beginning to feel as if I'm part of the place. Outside my flat half a dozen girls are sitting around on a parapet gossiping. I imagine that this

161

is a version of the village well, where they would meet friends and exchange news. I can't think what they find to talk about, living in this enclosed world, but they never seem to be short of subjects. I just wish I could understand them. I might feel as if I'm getting to know people but I'd need to speak Amharic and live here for a long time *really* to know them. And even then I wonder how much I'd be accepted. Maybe I'm not so much a part of their world after all.

Amina isn't in the ward. Some patients are sitting outside in the sun, gossiping. When I ask after her no one knows where she is. I'm walking back when I see her on the path coming towards me. Tears are streaming down her cheeks. My first instinct is to give her a hug, but I hesitate because I'm not at all sure if that would be culturally acceptable. Instead, I give her a pat on the shoulder. Of course I know that she doesn't understand English; still, I foolishly ask, 'What's the matter? Are you all right?'

She stares at me dumbly then looks down at the ground. She's wearing cheap plastic shoes, coloured pink. She raises one foot and turns the shoe upside down. It's full of urine.

Just then one of the nurses, Sister Wongelwit, comes along. Her name means Woman of the Gospel. I can never remember it, but she's told me that it's all right just to call her Gospel. She explains that Amina had the catheter removed yesterday, and since then she's been wet. She's also had abdominal cramps, for which she's been given drugs.

Poor Amina looks as though her heart will break. We take her to see Sister Belaynesh, the psychiatric nurse. She has a small office off to one side of the main entrance, which she shares with Sister Konjit. Belaynesh sits her down, holds her hands and they speak quietly together.

'This is the time when they need counselling,' Belaynesh tells me. 'She was expecting to be cured. She feels depressed and a sort of hopelessness. I'll counsel her and help her to accept the situation. It usually happens when the catheter is removed. The urethra is used to that catheter and it may not be simple to hold urine. But after a while things might settle down and she will improve. Sister Azeb will give her pelvic floor exercises to improve continence. Even if she doesn't get better straight away, she can go home and after a while she still might be all right. If she's not dry she can come back after six months and maybe we'll try another operation. She will improve. This is not the end of the road.'

Amina seems a lot brighter after talking to Belaynesh. She's decided to count her blessings. Both of her fistulas have been cured, and even though she's still wet it's nowhere near as severe as before.

Later that day Catherine sees Amina and gives me her assessment. 'She's a bit wet. There's a tiny bit of infection. We did a dye test and there's no hole. I've put the catheter back in and I'll take it out again in a few days. She could have a little bit of stress incontinence, but I'm sure she'll be all right.'

Next day I'm over at the Bethlehem ward again. Amina is sitting outside with some other women. There's a steady drip, drip, drip, falling to the ground beneath her. Nevertheless she smiles happily and waves. She appears to be over her depression.

Zemebech has also had a slight setback, according to Dr Abiy. It's day fifteen since her operation and the catheter was removed yesterday. She's dry but she's having what they call 'urgency'. Abiy explains that because she's been leaking continuously, the bladder's nervous system has been compromised. She doesn't know when she needs to go to the toilet, so she's been having some embarrassing accidents. It's a common outcome after surgery. After a time the nervous system will retrain itself and she'll return to normal. Just in case there's some other reason for her condition they'll test her for urinary tract infection. 'But really,' says Abiy, 'she's cured, and I'm happy with that.'

Judging from the big smile on her face, Zemebech is pretty happy too.

Now to Halema, the Somali patient, about whom Dr Biruk was so pessimistic. It's fifteen days after her operation and she looks happy for the first time. We have the usual language problem, so I have to hear from Dr Biruk how she is. He tells me she's doing fine. She's still dry. He plans to clamp the catheter today and that will tell him if her continence mechanism is functioning. If she's dry they'll take it out tomorrow. Removing the catheter will be the big test.

The last time I saw Alganish she was doing well. I'm looking forward to catching up with her. She is so determinedly optimistic and uncomplaining that I've developed a bit of a soft spot for her.

I remember that Dr Mulu was worried that she could develop stress incontinence. As always, Alganish has a happy smile and seems glad to see me. I hold her callused hand and, with the ward sister translating, ask how she is.

The news is not good. She's wet. Her card says that she's leaking and there's a slight sloughing of the wound. I feel a rush of sadness, which takes me by surprise. It's as if this misfortune is happening to a member of my own family.

Mulu isn't around so I ask Catherine for her opinion. She thinks Alganish's fistula has healed and that she's just leaking around the catheter. The leaking isn't a concern, but the sloughing is. Catherine had a patient just like this recently and the repair broke down. They'll need to keep the catheter in for another week and see how she progresses.

Catherine's verdict: she's half-cured.

When I last saw Leteabazgi she was in the recovery ward having just had her operation. She was feeling pretty awful then. Dr Biruk did the operation, and it was a difficult one. A big defect, combined with a short urethra, makes her a prime candidate for stress incontinence. Five days after the operation she developed cramps in the abdomen which gave her a lot of pain. It's now eight days and she's doing well. D, d and d. For the first time since I met her she looks happy.

The other Lete, Letelibanes, has had a dream recovery. The catheter was removed yesterday and she's perfectly dry. She's getting ready to go home tomorrow.

Next day I get up at 5 am to see her off. It's still pitch-dark at that time of day. A group of nine women and four men are waiting in the car park. I presume that the men are relatives. Letelibanes is there, wearing a pretty green dress with her plastic bag of belongings over her shoulder.

The driver, Hamid, arrives with a coat thrown on over his pyjamas. He shares a *tukul* with one of the other drivers in the compound. He stretches, rubs his eyes, starts the Toyota Troopy and we all pile in. I sit in the front and everyone else squashes together on the two long bench seats in the back. I tell Hamid that there's room for a couple more in the front. 'No problem,' he replies. The *ferenji* gets special treatment, apparently.

There's a festive feeling in the car. A bit of pushing and shoving as they all try to squeeze in. Lots of joking and giggling. And why wouldn't there be? These women have all been through an agonising labour, followed in some cases by years of rejection, and now they're cured and off to new beginnings.

The Toyota does a three-point turn and a patient is caught in the headlights, with her shawl wrapped around her against the cold. She's got out of bed to say goodbye to a friend. She lifts her hand and waves, and we sweep up the drive into the early morning streets.

The bus station is a huge area, covering acres of ground; even at this time of day it's seething with people. I wonder how those who don't speak Amharic and can't read could find the right bus. But then, they find their way here from far-flung corners of the country, so I suppose they can find their way back home.

For such a momentous occasion everything happens quickly and without ceremony. The car pulls up, the passengers get out, say a brief goodbye and disappear into the crowd. I give Letelibanes a wave, she smiles and waves back, and she's gone.

A lot has been happening while I've been away. Sister Belaynesh has a patient who's psychotic. She's a middle-aged lady from Oromo province. She's been getting out of bed and wandering around complaining that people are sticking needles into her – not just an injection, she thinks she's being attacked. Ruth Kennedy noticed her and asked one of the Oromo sisters, Mulenesh, to come and pray with her. 'That settled her right down, then I gave her some Valium and she calmed down. But she'll get sick again. It just takes a while. They behave like that for two or three days and then they'll come out of it.'

After the operation everything's so strange for some patients that they get quite psychotic and they're totally unaware that they're behaving irrationally. Sister Belaynesh usually gives them Largactyl or Valium and lets them sleep, then after a while they come good.

★

I pay a visit to Catherine in her house to catch up. Yeshi brings in a tray with a pot of her super-strength coffee and some snacks. I'm pleased to see Gordon's Prince Charles biscuits are still holding out. Also on the tray are half a dozen cheques for Catherine to sign. She still hasn't got used to how much money they are spending these days. 'We have to pay out a tremendous amount each month,' she says. 'There's millions of dollars around. Clive Hewitt, the head of the trust in Britain, keeps saying, "I don't know why this money keeps rolling in to me each week."'

Catherine is worried because all of the trusts are being run by old people now. Clive is in his seventies. Stuart Abrahams, who runs the Australian trust, is also in his seventies. After fourteen years working for the hospital, he's grooming a younger man to take over.

'They've mostly been volunteers,' Catherine says. 'We were paying Stuart a little to begin with, then he said, "I can't get a pension if I'm being paid and I can get more from the pension than you can pay me." Clive pays one man – a friend of his – a pittance, really, to go into the office three days a week.

'In America we have to pay Kate Grant. She has to have a salary. I don't know about the other trusts. The Swedish one has a lot of women parliamentarians in it.'

When Catherine first came to Ethiopia her salary, paid by the government, was 1400 birr per month. Reg earned 1800. That was about $400 Australian, between them. 'We lived on that for many years. You could live very cheaply then. You couldn't live on that now.'

The government still pays her a salary, only it's gone up to 2000 birr a month. 'I've still got a contract which they renew every three years. I was supposed to retire at 55. I'm about 30 years overdue. When I'm 85, if I survive, it'll be 30 extra years that they've been paying me a contract. If they keep renewing it, that is.' She also earns a small salary from the Ethiopian trust.

Catherine's current concern is pigs. It seems that some of the staff at Desta Mender have been raising pigs and selling them, and Catherine's not happy about it. 'They've all got these wretched pigs out there and they're making money with them. And the pigs live right beside our fence. I told them we can't have pigs next to a hospital. How can you work with pigs when you're Orthodox? Orthodox or Muslims don't touch pigs. And they're making money. They're selling them to the supermarkets.

'I said they can work the pigs if they have them well away from the compound edges. They have them right down at the bottom of the paddock, not on the inside, but outside. I think they're all in it. We can't stop them from doing it, but we have to be sure they're not taking grain from the horses and giving it to the pigs. They could be doing that.'

One of Catherine's greatest concerns about all this expansion is that the hospital will lose the family atmosphere which has made it so special. 'I think I've got a very good staff but I don't know them all now. I know all the sisters, but it's difficult for me to know all the little nursing aides. Yesterday in the ward I said to Matron, "It's hard to do our work, there are so many of them." I found two of them sitting behind a bed – they didn't know what to do, they were sitting on the floor. She said three of them are going up to Andrew, at Bahar Dar, and a lot of them will go to Harar when it opens. They should go to the centres now and learn how to run a centre. So we're going to do something about that.

'It's difficult to keep the family spirit going. We're having some problems with staff. There was a little fighting in the theatre the other day, for instance. Some new nursing aides were being rude to the senior nursing aides. Things like that [are] going on. It's very difficult to keep everyone happy. They've all got family worries and complaints about their salaries. The cost of living's going up here. I think it's just so big that it's difficult to keep it all in the same atmosphere.

'We had a stormy management meeting yesterday when Ephraim [the manager at Desta Mender] was talking about Desta Mender and all the problems there. There are a lot of things that need to be settled. We're just wondering about sending these girls off until they're trained. Ephraim is reluctant to send them until everything's settled. But people like Rosemary [Burke, the Englishwoman who is helping at Desta Mender for six months] think they should go.

'For instance, these two sewing girls – we're procrastinating [about] sending them down to Yirgalem [the fistula hospital in the south], because the house that they were going to rent has fallen through. The landlord reneged and said he didn't want to let it. So we have to find a new house. But they could go and live in the nurses' home that we're renting at the moment. I'm sure once they get down there they would find a house. They're grown-up people, really; they're used to living in a village. The decision was to send them.

'I don't see how these poor vegetable girls can set up a vegetable farm, for instance. I think we're getting a big lot of land, but it's still not certain. It's so tiresome. Poor old Ephraim is a bit overwhelmed, I think.'

I think Ephraim isn't the only one who sometimes finds it all a bit too much.

Catherine is concerned about one patient who speaks a very rare language, called Dimi. The Dimi people come from way down in the south of the country. There are so few of them that you'd never find a translator in Addis Ababa. They sometimes speak a language called Ari, which is used by an adjoining tribe. There are a lot more Ari, so Catherine had been hoping she'd be able to find one. Then she discovered that her patient doesn't speak Ari anyway. She's been here for a month and has been unable to speak a word to anyone. One of her ureters has become disconnected from the bladder. It was Catherine's operation and she thought she'd done a good job, but sometimes these things happen. 'It's easy to fix,' she says, 'but the poor woman thinks that her operation has been a failure and that she's not cured. No one can explain to her that she's going to be all right.'

Another of her worries is a seventeen-year-old girl upon whom she operated a couple of days ago. She'd had an emergency caesarean in a government hospital. Whoever did it removed her uterus and didn't tell her. Catherine's seen this happen often with inexperienced doctors. When they do a caesarean they sometimes think the uterus is gangrenous, when really it's ischaemic – that is, there's a lack of blood supply. The correct procedure is to leave it and allow it to repair itself. Instead they remove it, and in doing so they sometimes damage the base of the bladder, the trigone, causing a fistula as well.

Catherine is visibly angry. 'They do this all the time,' she says. 'They say they've got a ruptured uterus. But in all my years, here and at Princess Tsehai, I've never seen a primiparous woman [with her first child] with a ruptured uterus. It's an appalling thing to do, to rob a woman of her chance to be a mother and not even tell her. I had to tell this poor girl that she'll never be able to have children.'

A few years ago Dr Mulu received a phone call from a French doctor in Axum saying that he wanted to send them a patient. He'd performed a caesarean on her and removed a stillborn baby, along with her uterus, her ovaries and her bladder.

'Why did you do that?' asked Mulu.

'Oh, they were necrotic and ischaemic, I had to take them out. I've taken the ureters out to the stomach wall.'

'You've destroyed this woman's life,' said Mulu. 'Why are you calling us now?'

'Because I'm leaving.'

According to Ruth, who told me this story, it shows ignorance of Africa. A woman without a uterus is no one. She cannot have children, which is the chief reason for existence in her community. The uterus and other organs may look terrible but the correct procedure is to close the patient up and leave it. The uterus has great powers of regeneration. If it sloughs off, then let it, she will pass it naturally. But when it's gone the woman is ruined. She's no longer a woman in the eyes of her community.

Ruth has also been having difficulties. A doctor and a nurse, both women, have arrived from Afghanistan for a month's training. They're staying in the guest house and Ruth has had to find food for them, prepared the Muslim way, and a Muslim cook.

Dr Forzana Wali Jebran and her nurse, Monisa Dostdar, are from a hospital in Kabul which is funded with American money. They've seen many women with fistulas, but they've never been able to do anything about them because no one in Afghanistan can do the surgery.

Dr Forzana has been practising obstetrics for fourteen years. She was able to keep working all through the time of the Taliban, which probably says something about her character. She's quite mild-mannered, but underneath there's a steely resolve. This is someone who knows what she wants and is determined to get it. After having spent a couple of days in the theatre she's not happy with the progress she's making. She wants to do some operations and she wants to do them now! Also, she's heard that Andrew is a good teacher. She tells Ruth she must go to Bahar Dar, otherwise she won't learn anything.

When she gets her back up, Ruth Kennedy can be pretty formidable herself. 'She has to know that she can't come in here and make demands,' she thunders. She's writing her a note to let her know how the system works around here.

Dr Forzana was assisting Catherine in the theatre yesterday. Catherine is worried that she's a bit too bull-at-a-gate. She's told her that when she gets back home she must start with easy cases, otherwise she'll have failures and then no one will come to her.

There's also a problem finding a doctor for the new fistula hospital at Harar, which is due to open in six months' time. The surgeon at the government hospital who was offered the job has knocked it back. He can't afford it. He earns 30,000 birr a month; their doctors only get half that.

'They sacrifice a lot to work here,' says Ruth Kennedy.

Ruth, like Catherine, is a staunch champion of the Ethiopian staff. During recent pay-scale deliberations it was decided that eight senior staff, including all the doctors, would be given cars. The doctors were asked what sort of cars they would like. They conferred and decided upon a Honda four-wheel drive. A couple of weeks later they came back and said they'd discovered that the Nissan was $6000 cheaper. That would save the hospital $48,000. So they asked for the Nissan.

This is precisely why, Ruth contends, this hospital will continue to prosper through this period of change. The staff regard it as more than just a job; they're committed to its welfare.

Just then Catherine walks in. She wants to discuss a situation in Bahar Dar. One of the guards has been sleeping with a nurse aid. They found out and dismissed the guard. Catherine is very annoyed. 'It's not up to us to moralise like that. Why just the guard? It was good that the girl, who has a stoma, found someone to fall in love with. It would have been better to encourage them to go and get married.'

Ruth will investigate. It happened while Andrew was away;

they suspect it might have been the matron – who's a bit of an authoritarian – who fired the guard.

It turns out to be a misunderstanding. The guard had not been dismissed, but had simply left to live outside, after living in the compound. He and the nurse aide married and are living together. They both still work at the hospital.

Ruth tells Catherine that she's received encouraging news about little Sayed in Holland. Tests have shown that she suffered no damage from the overdose of oxygen. She'll be on her way home soon.

That night we're having dinner at Catherine's place. She shows not the slightest sign that the day-to-day problems are weighing her down. She's positively lighthearted. She launches into a story about giving the driver, Daniel, a letter to post to Stuart Abrahams in Sydney that morning. She was about to put the stamps on when she noticed that they showed pictures of Surma women from the south of Ethiopia, with naked breasts. 'I took the letter back and asked Daniel to find a more suitable stamp. I was worried about the effect the stamps would have on Stuart.'

Ruth and I burst into laughter. Catherine, I suspect, is well aware of the effect she has with these quirky little tales, and she laughs happily along with us. She says she's thinking of sending one to my wife, Anna, with a note saying that these are the people John's hobnobbing with.

Her sense of fun is infectious. The talk over dinner turns to presents. Ruth was walking from her house to her office this morning when she heard someone calling, 'Sister Hirute Kennedy. Sister Hirute Kennedy.' It was a former patient, lugging a big plastic jerrycan. She'd travelled three days by bus with this 30-kilogram jerrycan full of honey to give to the staff.

Ruth's housegirl, Berhani, and an assistant had spent the entire day decanting it into containers for distribution.

Catherine has received many strange presents over the years. She was once doing a clinic in outpatients when a grateful patient presented her with a chicken. She placed it on the end of the examination table, thinking that she and Reg would have it for dinner that night. Then it laid an egg. It proved to be such a good layer that its demise was postponed for a couple of weeks.

I've tried hard to avoid using the word 'saint' in relation to Catherine Hamlin. It gets used a lot when people write about her in newspapers, and on TV. She dislikes it. It embarrasses her to be called a saint, but it's hard to dampen the enthusiasm of her admirers. It's true to say that Catherine does what she does, for God. She'd prefer to do it in complete anonymity, except that she has to raise money. And for that, she realises that the best commodity she has to sell is herself. Journalists will write what they want. Saint. It's an overused word, but I know why people resort to it. I myself have never met such an unquestionably good human being. Which makes what happens at the end of the evening extraordinary.

Just before we're leaving to go home to our beds, Catherine says in an offhand way that she sometimes wakes up at night worrying that she hasn't done enough to help. Worrying about how God will judge her when she gets to heaven.

CHAPTER 17

Most days I take an hour off and go for a walk outside the hospital. Living within the walls of the compound begins to feel a little surreal after a while; I need to get away now and then to remind myself what the rest of the world is like.

Walking towards the main gate I notice a solitary patient crouching like a bird on a seat. She has pulled her shawl over her head so that it hides her face. There's a puddle underneath her on the ground. She sits there motionless, eyes downcast, as though she's hiding from the world. Bereft, I think.

I go out the gate and up the hill past the building site where women work in pairs, carrying trays of rubble out to a pile on the road. Past the fruit stall where they charged me twice the proper price for bananas. Past people waiting at the bus stop.

On the corner there is a cluster of ramshackle stalls and four or five beggars all in a row. I give some coins to an old, crippled man. I turn left and walk along the main road. The exhaust fumes are bad today. I wonder what they do to the health of those beggars and the vendors who work perpetually in their stink.

There's a section of about 100 metres where a corrugated iron fence hides another building site. The man with the grossly swollen legs is crouched halfway along as usual. He sits perfectly still, staring straight ahead, with his trousers pulled up to show his lower limbs. His feet and ankles look like bags of liquid. Ruth, who knows everything, tells me that his disease is called podoconiosis, or 'mossy foot'. It's caused by tiny particles of silica in the soil penetrating the skin and causing lymphatic obstruction. It results in similar problems to those from elephantiasis. Prevention is just a matter of wearing shoes and using soap. Simple. Or maybe not so simple. He's always there in the same spot – a young man, no older than his mid-twenties. I've never seen him move or acknowledge another person. Not even when I give him a coin.

Further along I pass the Shell service station, where the Shell Shop is, curiously, a dry cleaners. I come to a cluster of shops and vendors with their goods displayed on mats on the ground. There are piles of cheap socks, underwear, clothing. One man has rows and rows of shoe liners for sale. A woman with a baby in her lap offers those little straps that attach to computer memory sticks. I wonder, how many of those would she sell?

There are numerous shoe-shine boys. They are among the few who seem to do a brisk trade. Each one, usually a young boy, squats in the dirt with a can of water and a rag to clean the shoes, and an assortment of brushes and polish, usually kept in a tattered bag. Each has a chair for the customer and a little wooden stand for them to rest their foot. It doesn't require a big capital outlay to be a shoe-shine boy.

There's always one man with a pile of broken watches for sale. Why would anyone buy such junk? Others are selling sunglasses. A boy sits like a statue, his oustretched hand draped with cheap necklaces. I pass a child of about six, standing patiently beside a weighing machine, and 50 metres further on, another. There are three or four people with wheelbarrows full of lemons. They must have just come into season, for I have not seen lemons here before.

The beggars are thick in this part. I count ten in the space of 100 metres. Even begging is a competitive business. There are two or three very old men, a blind man sitting patiently with one hand held out, worrybeads on the other wrist. A couple of women sitting in the dirt with filthy children. An old leper woman whose fingers have been entirely worn away. She has two knobs where her hands should be. Another leper, a man, with a disfigured face. A couple of cripples, one sitting on the ground with two shrivelled, bare legs thrust out in front of him. His feet are tiny and turned in so that the toes face each other. There are lumpy calluses on the sides. A few clothing and footware stores. A shop selling beauty products.

People of all classes make their way through this throng. Bush boys with bare legs and muddy sandals, blankets thrown over their shoulders, carrying staffs. A man leading a herd of donkeys carrying bags of grain to market. Men and women dressed in clean western clothes. An Orthodox priest with his black soutane and square-topped hat. A woman swathed in pink. She's wearing sandals, and I notice that the edges of her feet have been inked with an intricate design.

The vendors spruik for custom. At the roundabout which goes under the overpass, hordes of blue-and-white mini-buses are gathered, the conductors shouting their destinations. Here and there some grubby blankets, a few battered cooking things, show where people have made their homes.

I give money to the old leprous woman and to one of the men. I can't give to all. It's like the Fistula Hospital. It cures some people and it fails to cure others. And all over the country there are tens of thousands of fistula sufferers who will never even have the chance to be cured. They do what they can. They can't fix the whole problem – I can't fix the whole problem –

there is a much wider solution required for that. But you can help fix some of it.

An hour later, back inside the walls, I'm struck, as always, by the contrast. Peace. Cleanliness. Hope. No wonder some patients are reluctant to leave.

The bereft woman has not moved. She is still alone.

Ruth is having some visitors from Alaska to lunch. Dr Nell Wagonner, her teenage daughter and her daughter's friend. Dr Wagonner is another fistula convert. She trained in Addis. She's on her way home after working in Sierra Leone, and already she can't wait to return to Africa. She tells us about the situation in Sierra Leone; then the conversation turns to a pipeline which is being built in Alaska to carry gas to the rest of mainland USA. It has aroused the anger of conservationists. 'Why?' Catherine wants to know. She uses 'why' a lot. 'Why will a pipeline make a difference to the environment?'

Dr Wagonner explains that it's all the disruption that will be caused during the construction that's the problem. Catherine wants to know all the details. What sort of disruption? What sort of animals are affected? What about polar bears? Are there many left in Alaska? Are they in danger? Why? What? Where? She has the eagerness of a twenty-year-old.

At these informal social occasions Catherine often mentions, in a kind of jocular aside, that she's getting old. 'I probably won't be around much longer,' she says brightly. She explains to Dr Wagonner's daughter that she has lymphoma, which could carry her off suddenly at any time. 'The good thing about lymphoma is that it acts quickly in old people. Don't get cancer when you're young,' she advises. 'It acts much more slowly.'

After having brought up her impending demise, she quickly changes the subject. 'Any rate, that's enough about that.'

★

Ruth has solved the problem of the troublesome Afghani ladies. Einar Lande, the Norwegian doctor who runs the new hospital at Yirgalem, has gone home on leave, so Dr Mulu is going down for a few days to do some operations. She's taking the Afghanis with her. They'll get some broad experience there with Mulu teaching them one-on-one.

Yirgalem is in the south. I'm heading in the other direction, north to the new hospital at Mekele.

CHAPTER 18

During three different trips to Ethiopia I've visited several large towns. Mekele is without doubt the most pleasant I've seen. It's clean and quiet. Traffic is sparse. The air is unpolluted. The streets are laid out in an easy-to-navigate grid pattern. It's the only place I've been where I can walk about without being accosted by hawkers or people hissing '*ferengi*' at me. There are no beggars. It's clearly a prosperous place. Mekele is in Tigray, which is known as a rich province. Tigray is where the Ethiopian Prime Minister, Meles Zenawi, comes from. Maybe that has something to do with it.

The fistula hospital at Mekele is an attractive, low building next to the government hospital. Everything looks new and well cared for. The surgeon in charge, Dr Melaku Abriha, is a big, comfortably built man with a gentle manner. He is courteous and friendly, and speaks fluent English. There are only half a dozen patients in the ward. The hospital has been open for sixteen months; it will take a while for people out in the countryside to hear about it. Dr Melaku isn't worried. He says the same thing happened at Bahar Dar in the beginning. It took about eighteen months for word to spread, and then they were inundated with patients. 'We're sure people are still hiding patients in the villages. Because this is a very fertile area, they concentrate on farming. They leave the lady in the cottage. She will be fed and given water and milk, that is all they can do for her during this planting period.'

An Ethiopian non-government organisation (NGO), the Relief Society of Tigray, has been finding patients for them in the southern region. They transport them to the hospital and give them an allowance of 30 birr per day, for fifteen days, while they stay. It's a great incentive for the patients. Most of them get cured and they have some money as well to help them become re-established in society.

At first the NGO brought in a lot of patients who turned out not to have fistulas at all. Dr Melaku trained their nurses how to identify fistulas by doing dye tests. That proved to be successful, so the NGO is now going to expand their activities to the western region. As well as that, Dr Melaku is hiring an outreach coordinator who will go out into the villages and spread the word.

One thing that helped raise awareness was a broadcast on local radio about a couple of the hospital's early cases – a mother and daughter who both had fistulas.

Dr Melaku was first attracted to fistula surgery when he did his postgraduate studies in Addis Ababa. After having worked in government hospitals, Addis was a revelation to him. 'When you go in you don't think you are in Ethiopia. In government hospitals there are a lot of problems – budget levels, lack of commitment. Everybody stops for a long tea break, then at twelve noon they start getting ready to go home for lunch. Everything stops, patient evaluation, whatever is going on. You get your lunch and take coffee, then when you return you're tired, so you stay for a few minutes then you run away for the afternoon break.

'In the Addis Fistula Hospital it was not like that. You work straight through, have a few minutes for lunch, a few minutes for a break, all within the hospital. It is amazing. Even sometimes you'll miss your lunch but that's okay. By the time it's 4 pm everything is settled in the hospital for the day, and you feel satisfied. As a physician I wanted to be a part of this thing some day.'

Dr Melaku's teachers were Catherine, Ambaye and Mamitu. His introduction to fistula surgery included, inevitably, Mamitu's infamous dye trick. She sprung it on him during an outreach trip to Metu government hospital at the end of a particularly long and trying day's surgery, without pause for lunch. He still chuckles every time he thinks of it.

He did 26 simple cases whilst training, then got a job as a gynaecologist at Adigrat Hospital in the north-east of the country. The two gynaecologists before him had both been interested in fistula surgery. One had stayed for five years and the next for seven, so there'd been twelve years of continuous service for fistula patients. The hospital even had a dedicated fistula ward with twelve beds.

Dr Melaku continued the service although, without special operating tables, special sutures and instruments, it was difficult doing the surgery. He did straightforward cases, and the hard ones he referred to Addis Ababa. He began to appreciate some of the peculiarities of this little-known branch of obstetrics. 'Fistula surgery is different from other surgery. Patients need not only medical treatment, they need psychological support, love and sympathy. Most of them are stigmatised, so you have to be very sympathetic.

'You have to be patient also. In fistula surgery you see your result after weeks, not straight away. With a hysterectomy, if you do it properly you know your patient will be okay after anaesthesia. You fear anaesthesia in normal surgery. Here the fear is, will she be dry or not? So you suffer with the patient for weeks. It's not for everyone – you need commitment. And after going through a lot of difficulties, when a patient is cured the reward is huge.'

In the time that he's been at Mekele, Dr Melaku has seen some curious cases. None more curious than that of a deaf patient from a village near Axum. Zewdi became deaf at the age of four or five, following a disease – probably meningitis. Unable to communicate, she led an isolated life. She was an only child. Her mother was worried, because in a place where girls are married at thirteen and fourteen, she had reached the age of 28 with no husband. Fearing for the family line, she arranged with a neighbour, a married man with four children, to visit her daughter secretly at night and impregnate her. She promised him that she would tell no one about it and would not ask for a penny to help raise the child.

It was nothing less than sanctioned rape. Dr Melaku shakes his head in disbelief when he talks about it. 'Imagine the feelings when she had to go with this married man. She was a virgin. He visited her more than once, probably – they had to see that she was pregnant. It would have been a big issue if it had been made public in the village; the man would not have acknowledged the child. Because of what her mother did she was almost wrecked.'

Remarkably, they managed to keep the pregnancy a secret. Zewdi's mother apparently believed that after the baby was born, her daughter would be able to stay inside all the time and avoid going to the market, or any place where she would meet people. The plan was never put to the test, for she had an obstructed labour, the baby was born dead and the daughter was left with a fistula.

The whole bizarre business – the secret visits, the hidden pregnancy, long labour, the tragic aftermath – happened without anyone in the village knowing about it. It was only when an uncle was visiting and noticed the smell that the story came out. Wisely, he brought Zewdi to the hospital. The mother was too ashamed to come.

This hapless young woman had a big effect on everyone who cared for her. Her disability was bad enough, her mother's betrayal was scarcely believable, but then to cap it all she had ended up with a fistula. Cursed not once, but three times. Everyone's heart went out to her.

She was a model patient, always willing and uncomplaining. Dr Melaku recalls that when she tried to communicate she made sounds, but no one could understand them. Still, 'She understood we were doing our best for her and she accepted whatever we did.'

The operation was a complete success. Zewdi's uncle came to collect her and as she said goodbye they saw what they had all been waiting for. She was smiling.

On the ward round Dr Melaku treats each patient with grave courtesy. He studies the notes carefully, makes his examination and closely questions the nursing sisters. The ward is spotlessly clean. The floors gleam, the windows are unblemished by so much as a smudge. The staff's uniforms are blindingly white. After finishing the round we retire to his little office off to one side of the main entrance. There is not a speck of dust anywhere. His laptop computer and his pens and pencil sharpener are positioned with geometrical exactness on the desk top. This is a man who is rigorous in his approach to his profession. You could be excused for thinking that he's a bit of a martinet, but then out of nowhere he reveals his soft side.

We're chatting away easily when I casually ask him what he thought of Dr Hamlin when he first met her. He pauses for a long moment without saying anything, then two big tears well up. After what seems an eternity he manages to speak. 'Oh, I don't have any word to express that feeling. She is an angel.'

He has to pause again to wipe his eyes. 'Still operating too,' I say rather inanely. It's more to give him time to recover than an attempt at real conversation.

He manages a choking reply. 'Yes, still operating.'

When he has regained his composure he continues. 'Dr Hamlin is not Ethiopian. She and her husband came for a short term and they saw these patients all suffering from fistula. People like them are the people who make a difference in the world. They have a great place in everyone's heart. This is the strength that makes me want to work here.'

Sentiment aside, Dr Melaku is in awe of Catherine's clinical abilities. 'Whenever she's around she makes a difference. When you make a round with her she knows every patient. Her instinct is amazing. When she examines a patient she sees immediately if there's a problem. Late in the afternoon when everyone's getting ready to go home, she looks around and she solves a lot of problems which have not been detected during the whole day. I feel that she has an instinct for patients. She prays for her patients, and that's good. If you start to work for her it's difficult to withdraw from this system.'

Like everyone else, Dr Melaku is troubled by the thought of a future without Catherine Hamlin. It's not the fund-raising, or the management, or even the medical side that worries him. It's something less definable. 'She has been there for quite a long time, with the patients and staff and system all linked with her. She has founded everything, produced a lot of fistula surgeons, raised a lot of money. The money part and the skill and everything else can be replaced. But when Dr Hamlin goes, the hospital loses her spirit. The hospital will be functional, but her spirit – you can never replace that.'

I like Dr Melaku. And his colleagues in Addis. Every time I hear their stories I marvel at Catherine's good fortune at having gathered such remarkable people around her.

★

Back in Addis I see Mulu, who has returned from her stint in Yirgalem. She has discovered a problem there. Half the patients she saw had had caesareans in one of the hospitals in the area. The gynaecologist only comes there three days a week. On the other four days they're done by a general practitioner who's had a bit of O&G training. He's been cutting the top off the bladder, leaving the patients with very small bladders which are difficult to repair. Another bit of butchery to add to all the other butchery that happens in these places.

On the brighter side, the Afghani trainees have been able to do some surgery and they're happy. So that's one less problem to worry about.

CHAPTER 19

One of the most heartwarming events at the Addis Ababa Fistula Hospital has always been going-home day. Patients who have been cured are given their new dress and bus fare for the journey back to their village. Until recent times this little ceremony used to take place once a week in the main ward. It always included the 'dance of joy'. Proudly wearing their clean new dresses, the smiling patients would dance to the rhythm of clapping hands. Patients who were still recovering looked on with delight, no doubt imagining themselves celebrating in the same way before long. There were kisses and hugs, broad smiles, and often tears. Sometimes the women would want to kiss Catherine's feet. 'I love you next to God,' one once said. Then, with their fare in hand, they would be driven to the bus station, where they would depart to take up their new lives. There are so many patients now that the ceremony no longer happens, but the tradition of a new dress and bus fare home still remains.

As mentioned earlier, the hospital claims a 92 per cent success rate for fistula surgery. But of those 92 per cent, 30 to 35 per cent will still not be completely dry, due to lingering urinary incontinence. The hospital usually gives them three to

six months before deciding on further medical intervention. Dr
Biruk, who has made incontinence his specialty, says a fair guess
is that 15 per cent will come back after that time. The woman
may be dry when she is lying down, but when she stands up
or moves about, or perhaps when she coughs or laughs or lifts
something heavy, the urine runs out. Urinary incontinence,
which the doctors generally refer to as stress incontinence, is
the last obstacle left to overcome. As Andrew Browning puts
it, 'We're very good at closing the hole. But making people
continent by reconstructing all the continence mechanisms is a
completely different matter. And that's the challenge of fistula
surgery.'

Reg and Catherine Hamlin became aware of the problem
very early on. As long ago as 1967 they persuaded an eminent
Australian urologist, Dr Bob Zacharin, to come to Ethiopia to
consult. The day Dr Zacharin arrived, Reg picked him up at the
airport. Instead of taking him to his hotel to recover from the
journey, he drove him straight to the hospital in his VW. There
Dr Zacharin had to stand in the middle of a circle of patients
who were jumping up and down to see if there was any urine
on the floor.

Dr Zacharin had pioneered an operation which was successful
in Australia and other countries. But he was pessimistic about
being able to help these Ethiopian patients. Their condition
had been caused by traumatic injuries due to childbirth, which
would never happen to women in a developed country. They
had the added complication of scar tissue formation, especially
involving the urethra, the tube from the bladder to the outside.
This stiff, scarred urethra usually made the standard procedures
a failure.

Despite the disappointment, Bob Zacharin became a great
friend of the hospital. Under Reg and Catherine's instruction,
he learnt fistula surgery and went on to write a well-regarded

textbook on the subject. For many years he was a tireless fund-raiser and often used to visit, bringing with him medical equipment which had been slightly used and would otherwise have been thrown away. He always managed to talk his way through Customs, once joking that a bag of catheters was a new sort of spaghetti!

In 1995, a young Australian doctor, Judith Goh, was completing her specialty training as an obstetrician/gynaecologist. In her final year she had the option to work as a resident wherever she wanted to. Her sister was married to a surgeon, whose father, Barry Hicks, was a missionary doctor in Sodo, in southern Ethiopia. Judith elected to spend six months working in the hospital there. She met Catherine, and when her time in Sodo ended she spent a month in Addis Ababa learning fistula surgery.

Even after her sojourn in Addis she thought of fistula surgery as just a minor sidetrack on her chosen career path. She never imagined that she would become involved. Two years later, in 1997, Catherine asked her to come back to do a locum, as Dr Mulu was having a baby. It was then that the fascination took hold. 'I noticed that with a lot of women you closed the hole but they would not believe they were dry because they had such terrible incontinence.'

Although there were more than 150 different operations for stress incontinence, and more were being developed all the time, none was suitable for these Ethiopian women. Back in Australia, Judith discussed the problem with a Melbourne urogynaecologist, Marcus Carey, and together they began looking for a solution.

The urethra is one of the most wonderful and mysterious organs in the female body. It's only about 3.5 centimetres long, yet no one understands exactly how it works. It's basically a muscle that opens and closes, but there are a lot of little muscles and ligaments and support mechanisms that make it do what it does. When these components have been destroyed, it's easy enough to make an anatomical urethra – basically a tube – but to make a urethra that's functional is pretty well impossible.

An important part of the mechanism is the pubocervical fascia, which is a kind of sling, or hammock, which supports the urethra. At times of intra-abdominal pressure the urethra falls against this sling, the two walls of the urethra close and the urine stays in the bladder. It's a bit like stepping on a garden hose. With fistula patients, prolonged labour has often destroyed the pubocervical fascia, so instead of the hose encountering hard ground, the ground is soft and it will not close.

The most common procedure to fix incontinence is called the TVT operation. TVT, or tension-free vaginal tape, is a synthetic tape that goes underneath the urethra without tension, like a sling. At times of increased abdominal pressure the urethra falls against the tape, the walls close and the woman remains continent.

Right away the two Australians decided that the TVT was not suitable for the third world. One reason was that the tape then cost about $600. Also, the patients were going to have potential problems for the next 30 years. Living in the remote countryside they might not be able to access medical help if they needed it.

The answer was to make a *biological* sling. They make a sling from the cover, or fascia, that covers the muscles of the abdomen. They then make two small tunnels on the right and left side of the urethra, pass each end of the sling through these tunnels and fix them in place. Also, the urethra that is stuck behind the back of the pubic bone is mobilised during the procedure to make it more functional. Then a fat graft is placed between the back of the pubic bone and the freed urethra, to reduce the risk of the urethra adhering again.

In 2000 Judith and Marcus came to Addis Ababa to do a pioneer study. They operated on nine women and sent them home with a promise of money if they came back for followup examinations. Fourteen months later, seven of the nine returned. Six of them were dry – a result which made Judith very excited. 'Even if the two that didn't show up were not successful, still, six out of nine were happy. In Australia with simpler cases we tell patients that there's an 85 per cent chance of success, never 100 per cent.'

Judith and Marcus published a paper on their new operation, and in the 1990s and early 2000, papers were also published by one or two others who had become interested in the problem. Dr Biruk had taken a close interest in the new technique and since 2000 he has done the operation many times. His results have been a 70 per cent general improvement, but a complete cure has only a 40 per cent chance.

On the face of it, it seems that biological slings are not as good as the synthetic ones, which have a success rate in the range of 90 to 95 per cent; but this is in the west, where the pathology is quite different from that of patients in Ethiopia. With fistula patients there's the added factor of gross pelvic floor injury, due to such a traumatic childbirth. The fact is, no one really knows if the synthetic slings would give similar results with fistula patients. And no one knows, either, what the long-term prognosis is for the biological sling, because the patients just won't keep coming back.

Before doing the operation, Biruk does a urodynamic test. A year ago the hospital bought a $20,000 machine for the purpose. It gives a picture of the functional ability of the bladder and the urethra by measuring such things as how much the bladder holds, the change of pressure when there's a change in volume, the change in the pressure of the urethra during filling of the bladder, and other factors.

Biruk and one of the nursing sisters, Sister Genet, went to Germany to learn how to use the machine. In some cases – for instance, when the bladder is too small – there's no point at all in doing the operation. The machine tells them which patients are suitable. 'Before the machine came we were operating on all patients invariably,' says Biruk. 'Then we waited to see what would happen. Now we know exactly what to expect. We know those with a high possibility of cure, and we know when there's a 50 per cent or so cure rate, and we also know the patients for whom there's no point in operating.'

If the problem is a small bladder, there are things the doctors can do. The bladder can stretch with time, so they give it a few months. Or they can augment it by utilising tissue from organs such as the intestine to increase the size.

But this has its own problems. The gastro-intestinal tissue doesn't work the same way as bladder tissue. It cannot contract in the same way, so the method of pushing the urine out is not as efficient. The patient has to press on her abdomen or pass a catheter, so there may be some residual urine, or sometimes infection or stricture on the site where they put the new organ; the area can stenose, or narrow.

Another possibility is that of lengthening the urethra, using tissue from elsewhere in the body. But once more there are difficulties. One: because it's not proper urethral tissue, it doesn't really work like urethral tissue. It tends to be like a rigid pipe, so most of the time they can't achieve the sphincter capacity of the urethra. Another problem is a tendency of stricture – again, because it's not normal urethral tissue that's being used. What keeps a urethra from scarring is that it is lined with a mucosa, similar to the lining in the mouth. Without that tissue there is a tendency towards stricture. Biruk has seen it happen often. 'You discharge them and after some time they come back with a stricture. You have to dilate them, insert a catheter and so on, then reopen the site and do another procedure.'

It's only in the last three or four years that fistula surgeons have begun taking an interest in incontinence. Before, research had only been done by westerners such as the Hamlins, Judith Goh, Marcus Carey and a few others. In a sense, everything to do with stress incontinence in fistula patients is still pioneering medicine.

About four years ago Andrew Browning in Bahar Dar started looking for answers to the challenge. He, too, dismissed the TVT as being unsuitable for Ethiopia. Cost was a key factor. The tape now costs $900. 'My average cost is about $180 to $200 per patient for the whole three-week stay – meals, transport home, new dress, teaching, staff wages – everything.' He also worried about young women encountering problems with the tape years from now. 'I might move away, and who's going to be around to take them out? So I'd rather stay away from that.

'Ideally you want something here that can be easily replicated around Africa. If Dr Mwange is going to be working in a poor government hospital in Uganda, there's no way in the world they'll be able to afford synthetic slings. You want to have something that's quick and easy and is cheap and that works.'

After a lot of thought he came up with a new procedure. There are two muscles, called the pubococcygeal muscles, one on either side of the pelvis. He cuts each one along its length to make a flap, then joins the flaps together in such a way that they support the urethra. He has since found that even if there is no muscle remaining he can use any scar tissue that's left and get a good result. He now routinely uses this 'sling' with any fistula involving the urethra. The other important step is to take great care in maintaining the urethral length.

Andrew wrote a paper on his sling operation for the *British*

Journal of Obstetrics and Gynaecology. One of the referees pointed out to him that it wasn't entirely original. It was actually a variation of an old operation that had been used in the 1930s by two Polish surgeons, Ingleman and Suldeman. They had used the same tissue but in a different way. Their method would not be possible with Andrew's patients, as the obstructed labour causes too much tissue loss.

Andrew put an acknowledgment in his paper and it was accepted for publication. He claims his operation has pretty well halved the incontinence rate post-operatively. Still, the long-term outcome is unknown. At the time of writing there has been less than one year's followup. A doctor in Sierra Leone has done some and found that after six months or so the results were not so good.

If a patient is still wet after the sling operation, Andrew does a secondary procedure. It's predicated on the old-fashioned theory that urethral continence is a factor of its length and its width. He simply makes the urethra longer and thinner. He avoids the complications of using non-urethral tissues by using the bladder, tying it without cutting it, into the diameter of the urethra. With this procedure he has recorded about a 67 per cent complete cure rate. Even those who are not totally cured generally improve. Andrew cites the case of a patient who had been operated on six times previously. 'She was completely and hopelessly incontinent. I just made the urethra longer and thinner from the bladder, not at the vagina, because it never works, and she was completely cured.'

While these two different sling operations are producing partial success, the problem of incontinence is far from solved. In the developed world it's a whole sub-specialty. The urogynaecology training for incontinence is another three years on top of the six years for obstetrics and gynaecology, In Ethiopia, not one doctor has been trained in the specialty. Judith Goh believes that needs to change. 'They need to look into incontinence a bit more, not just the fistula operation. There's a whole list of reasons why women leak, and you need to do the right operation for the right person. That's what the training's all about, to pick when you do it and why you do it, not just how to do it.'

Judith believes that more research needs to be done into urge incontinence, which is the other main reason why fistula patients leak. Normally the bladder empties when a signal from the brain tells it to. With urge incontinence the signal doesn't get through, so it may empty at inappropriate times. There's no surgery for urge incontinence, and it is much more difficult to treat.

'Being a fistula surgeon is simple,' says Judith. 'There's a hole and you close it. There are techniques for different holes. Once you've got the skills you can do it. But looking at someone's quality of life, that's when you need to put a bit more thought into it. Why is she leaking? There are so many different reasons. If she's got a fistula she's leaking because she's got a fistula. The only option is surgery. But with incontinence, it's which surgery shall I do? And shall I do surgery to begin with?'

The mystery surrounding incontinence is just one of the unknowns with fistula patients. No one knows the long-term outcome for mental health. A joint survey by Judith in Bangladesh and Andrew in Ethiopia found there is a high risk of mental dysfunction with women before their fistula operation. That's hardly surprising, considering the life they've been leading. They did another survey recently, following patients immediately after surgery. If they're dry, then the risk of mental health dysfunction is the same as that of the general population. But they haven't been able to survey patients after they've gone home, to see how they reintegrate back into society. 'That is really what cure is,' says Judith, 'if they can go back and live in their community. We know there are a lot of problems, like sexual dysfunction. A lot of them are young women and they rely on falling pregnant; if the vagina is closed up that's not possible. So, will they be outcast again because they can't have children? A lot of them, because of psychological problems, or scarring in the uterus, might not have periods again, so there's a lot of reproductive dysfunction as well. There's a lot we don't know that's hard to find out.'

CHAPTER 20

Every couple of days I see a group of foreigners, led by either Ruth or Bethela Amanuel, doing a tour of the hospital. Bethela usually works in administration; she fills in whenever Ruth is not available. She speaks perfect English and everything she does, from making travel arrangements or organising the day-to-day movements of the car fleet, or showing visitors around, she does well. It's bright, educated young women like Bethela who will be vital to the future of this place.

You can tell what stage of the tour they're at from the visitors' demeanour. If it's just beginning, they look quite normal. Towards the end they'll have tears streaming down their faces. All sorts of people ask to be shown around. Often they'll be visiting medical professionals but, professional or not, no one is unaffected.

I know what they're feeling. During three decades in journalism, covering war and disaster, I saw more than the average share of human misfortune. When I was here in 2000 Ambaye had taken me on a tour of the ward. Stopping at each patient's bedside, she translated their stories for me. There were women who had been injured before their teens, a child who had sustained her fistula through being raped, women who had endured their injuries for decades, women who had been carried in close to death, women who were broken, traumatised, depressed . . . story after story of pain and rejection and shame. Halfway through the round I was choking back tears. Long before we had spoken to them all I had to call a halt. Ambaye told me that my reaction was quite normal.

The tour begins with a lecture in the meeting room at the administration building. The day I sit in, Ruth is in charge of a group of young women from Athens, Georgia, USA. One is a recent nursing graduate, another is studying something called childbirth aid, there's a midwife, a nutrition student, a pharmacy student and an older woman who is the mother of one of them. Six women from the richest country on earth, five in their late teens and early twenties, similar ages to many of the patients they will soon meet. Looking at their scrubbed faces, their clean, pressed clothes, I wonder how they could possibly visualise the life of their Ethiopian contemporaries. Of course, any thinking person living in a developed country must realise how privileged they are. These women know that life in Ethiopia is different. I wonder if they realise quite how different.

Ruth begins by telling them about obstructed labour, using a teaching model of a woman's abdomen with a baby-sized doll which fits inside. They listen attentively while she explains about the child being stuck in the birth passage through a malpresentation, or because of size. They probably know about this anyway – those studying medical subjects certainly would. It's when they hear that some women may be in labour for five or six days that the first signs of shock appear.

Then Ruth tells them about the life of a typical Ethiopian woman. At the age of two, she carries her first water jar. It's exciting for her because she's like her mum and big sisters. She gets to do all the fun things. A bit like us learning to cook or bake.

The audience nods, and Ruth continues.

By the age of eight she's carrying weight that most grown western women couldn't carry. She fetches all the water for the household, from anything up to 9 kilometres away; all the wood; all the eucalyptus leaves that are needed to keep the fire at the right temperature. When she's done that, she grinds the grain for *injera* – a never-ending job. In the northern regions they use a large stone with a small stone. When the grain has been ground it's sifted, then the bigger pieces are ground again and it's sifted again. If you feel these girls' hands they've got big calluses on their palms. In the south they use a mortar and pestle. There, the calluses are on the fingers. Their nails are concave from holding the mortar. They sing sometimes while they work, and sometimes they grind the grain together. The mortar and pestle method is probably less backbreaking than using the two stones.

When the flour is fine enough she puts it into a jar and mixes it with the water that she has carried from the well, then adds a little bit of starter batter from the previous batter to make it sour. She'll leave it for two or three days while it ferments, which increases the calories.

She spends a lot of time in her smoky kitchen. It's smoky because of the leaves she burns. She has a little fireplace made out of stones and there are three logs that she keeps moving in as they burn, then she adds the leaves to keep it at the right temperature. There's no chimney in the *tukul*. Because of the smoke, these girls often have upper respiratory infections; also eye problems.

When she's about nine, ten or eleven the girl's father will start looking for a husband for her. Amongst the Muslims it could be someone old enough to be her grandfather, but amongst the Orthodox it's usually a boy of sixteen or seventeen. Usually he'll be fully mature sexually. The families will get together and agree on a contract. A couple of goats, or maybe a cow, are exchanged for the daughter. There will then be a marriage ceremony, after which the girl will go and live with the young man's family.

She's not supposed to have intercourse until after her periods start. In most cases the mother-in-law looks out for her. She's been through the same thing herself. They've bought this girl, so she has some value. They don't want to spoil the goods too quickly. It's in the interests of the family to have healthy grand-children. Then, when she's deemed to be mature enough, she has sex and has her baby.

Because 54 per cent of Ethiopian children are stunted – boys more than girls, in fact – the girls' periods tend to come late, which is a protection for them. That's in the areas where the girls can be sexually active when young. Where they're circum-cised it's a different story. They're not able to have proper intercourse because their vagina has been sewn up until it's almost completely closed. They don't get pregnant very quickly, as it's hard for the sperm to get into the birth passage. If they do get pregnant the delivery is pretty traumatic.

Usually the girl has her period at about fourteen or fifteen, sometimes even later. Generally the initial period is a sort of preparatory one, and for the first year the girl doesn't produce much in the way of eggs. So the average age of delivery is around seventeen.

By now the Americans are visibly affected. You can see shock, resentment, incredulity, anger on their faces. Ruth cautions them not to be too judgmental. 'It's wrong for us to blame early marriage when in our own societies we're giving out condoms to fourteen-year-olds, so we have to be very careful,' she says.

The girl will go on working through her pregnancy. And

she'll continue working if she has a healthy baby. If the birth is normal she will stay in bed for six weeks. She takes care of her baby, she gets up now and then to have a bath, she's taken care of. They don't know quite what to do with someone who's had a stillbirth, but she's still allowed the six weeks. If the baby has been born dead and she ends up with a fistula, she'll lie on her sopping bed in a foetal position, turn her head to the wall, hoping that if she remains completely still she'll be okay. This is absolutely lethal. The muscles just shrivel up from disuse and she ends up with contractures of the hips and knees.

After the lecture has ended, the group is shown through the hospital and they hear some of the patients' stories. It's around about now that the first tears appear. I think it must be especially heartrending for women seeing what happens to other women who, simply through the randomness of fate, are handed the lives Ruth describes.

A few months before I came to Addis, Ruth had been on a journey to Chad taking home a patient who'd been at the hospital for more than a year. Arefa came from a nomadic tribe near the Sudanese border, far from any town. In order to keep their wealth, which is in cattle, in the family, her people traditionally intermarry their first daughters. Subsequent daughters can marry outside. Arefa had married her husband at the age of twelve. She very soon fell pregnant and went into prolonged labour, resulting in a double fistula and a dead baby. She was by then thirteen or fourteen.

Her family took her to a local hospital, where her mother stayed with her for an entire year. Her injuries were so shocking that nothing could be done in Chad to repair them. Eventually the UNHCR (the UN refugee agency) contacted the Fistula Hospital and asked if they would take her.

Ruth got in touch with some Swiss missionaries she knew in Chad and they agreed to pay for Arefa's trip. She came with her father – a typical nomad, who didn't speak the language and was bewildered by the bustling foreign city. He stayed for a month then went home.

Dr Ambaye was Arefa's surgeon. First off she had to do a colostomy to give her rectal defect time to heal. She then operated on the bladder fistula, then the rectal one, then the colostomy had to be reversed. Arefa had four operations over a period of a year.

After being away for so long she was very frightened about going back home. She had made friends at the hospital; she had forgotten her Arabic and spoke Amharic; being quite light-skinned she even looked like an Ethiopian. She was happy where she was. 'She actually asked to stay,' Ruth recalls, 'but we had no choice really, because we'd never have got her refugee status.'

There was a temporary reprieve when fighting broke out in Arefa's region. The hospital decided they'd better keep her where she was until the situation became safe.

The fighting ended. When it was time to go, Ruth contacted a missionary friend, Jill McKinnon, in Abeche, the nearest town to Arefa's family. Jill said she would be happy to look out for her. She offered to keep Arefa in Abeche and educate her.

Ruth spoke to Arefa's father and to a cousin of hers who was studying law in the capital, N'Djamena. She warned them that if Arefa went back to her husband it could kill her. 'I hear you,' the cousin said, 'but our elders may not understand.'

Ruth told him, 'If she goes back to her husband and she dies, before Allah it will be on your head. You're a lawyer; if I hear she's died I will never speak to your family again, I will believe you are people of two tongues.'

Arefa was delighted with her new life. She loved learning,

and she enjoyed living in a small town after the harsh nomadic existence she'd been used to. Always in the back of her mind was the worry that it might not last. Sure enough, after a few months had gone by, the elders of Arefa's tribe contacted Jill. They told her that Arefa needed to go out into the bush to spend a month with her family.

This was what Arefa had been dreading more than anything. She feared that they would force her to go back to her husband. She was still wet, and any sexual activity would have been extremely painful for her. Whether it could even have happened is doubtful because she was so badly scarred.

'Her father was looking after his interest,' says Ruth. She has asked Jill in Abeche to check up on Arefa. It's now three months since she went to see her family and she hasn't returned. 'That is a worry. There are people in Abeche who can look after her, but once you're out in the desert . . .' She shakes her head. 'Beautiful, beautiful girl . . .'

CHAPTER 21

The Fistula Hospital has had a long relationship with Chad, the landlocked desert nation which is said to be the poorest country in Africa. They've sent over surgical teams to do outreach clinics. The first time Andrew Browning went, he and Dr Haile and Sister Ruth Gadessa flew in a small plane across the Sahara Desert to a village next to the Sudanese border, near Darfur.

Some missionaries had collected about 40 patients for them. They operated in a tin shed in 50-degree heat. There was no air conditioning, not even a fan. Dressed in scrubs and working under hot theatre lights, they were dripping with perspiration. Andrew remembers going to his billet after a day's work, craving a shower. The thermometer was still showing 35, but after the OR it felt cold.

As tough as Andrew found it, his Ethiopian colleagues had the added burden of having to do without their cherished *injera*. As their assignment wore on, Haile would tick off the time remaining – 'Only nine days until *injera* . . . only eight days till *injera* . . . 'I don't know what it is about that stuff,' Andrew jokes. 'There must be something in it that's addictive.'

Many peasant people would probably spend their entire lives

without eating anything else, yet they still love it. I remember going to lunch with Catherine and Ruth and some visitors, to a rather smart restaurant in Addis Ababa. We invited our driver in to join us. The menu featured a range of dishes, from European to Ethiopian. Everyone chose European except the driver. Nothing could tempt him away from his usual *injera* and *wat*.

The next time a team went to Chad, it was to a different hospital. This time there was Andrew, Dr Haile and two nurses. When they turned up at Addis Ababa airport the Ethiopians were all carrying heavy bags. They were filled with enough ready-made *injera* to last them for two weeks; it must have been getting pretty stale towards the end.

The missionaries had put out a message on the local radio announcing that they were coming. By the time they arrived there were 40 or 50 patients waiting. One woman had travelled 100 kilometres across the desert on a donkey, after hearing on the radio that she could be cured. A French nurse, who was assisting them in the theatre, thought it would be nice to go back with her to her village to see how she fared. She wrote a letter to Andrew afterwards describing what had happened.

The patient had been a typical outcast, rejected by her husband and shunned by her friends and neighbours. She and the French nurse set off in a car together. By the time they reached the village, word had gone ahead that she had been cured. When she arrived, all the women who had previously rejected her welcomed her with gifts of food and perfume. The husband who had kicked her out had prepared a new bed for her and had even placed a new mat on the floor. The contrast after what she had endured previously was too much. She was so overcome that she wept tears of joy.

★

The surgeons do outreach trips to many different parts of Africa and Asia. They've been a few times to operate on the Mercy Ship, a hospital ship which travels up and down the west coast of Africa.

They sometimes go to other countries to teach. Andrew Browning believes this is the best way, because when people come to Addis to train they have all the specialised equipment, which they probably wouldn't have in their own setting. They have to learn to improvise. For instance, not all operating tables have a fold-away section at the end, so the surgeon may have to work sitting off to one side. Often the tables will not tilt enough, so they'll have to put cushions under the patient's bottom. If you get lots of blackouts you can put a caving light on your head. In one hospital in Uganda where Andrew taught, the steriliser was broken, so they just boiled up the instruments in a teapot.

'You can do a lot with very little resources. Doing medicine in developing countries, you realise how much the body heals itself. When to intervene, and how much to intervene, is a bit of an art. You can go overkill and do everything and the patient gets cured. Fair enough, but you're going to waste a lot of money and maybe even do the patient some damage, whereas if you just do a little bit and boost the patient along, eventually the problem will heal itself. Back in Australia, you see how tens of thousands more dollars get spent to increase the outcome by a tiny percentage. The bulk of medicine can be done with very little.'

Tucked away in obscure corners of Africa are people who have been doing fistula surgery for years with little recognition. Kees Waaldijk, a Dutchman, has done about 14,000 operations in Nigeria. He was originally a leprosy surgeon, doing things like tendon transplants and hand surgery. Then he saw the great need for fistula surgery. Although he wasn't an obstetrician/gynaecologist, he trained briefly in Addis, then pretty well made up his own techniques.

Kees is a tall man with grey hair and beard. He has big hands and a forceful personality. The first time Andrew Browning met him was in Geneva, where Andrew had gone to present a training manual that he'd written for the World Health Organization. Before even saying hello, Kees threw the manual on the table and declared, 'I don't agree with this at all.'

Two or three times a year Kees leaves his home and family in Holland and goes to Nigeria. He travels by car from hospital to hospital, usually operating on the same day that he travels. He does things which defy many of the basic rules of conventional surgery. He works without an assistant; he doesn't wear a cap or a mask; he doesn't use theatre lights, he simply pulls the table over to a window. He doesn't use drips; instead, he gets the patients to drink lots of water.

His surgical techniques are different from anyone else's. Everything is done in a minimalist manner. All fistula surgeons try to close the hole in such a way that there is no tension on the wound while it heals. The method pioneered by Reg and Catherine, which has become standard, is to mobilise the bladder – that is, to free it from surrounding tissue. They then close the hole with two layers of sutures and do a dye test to make sure the wound is watertight.

Kees achieves tension-free closure by doing minimal mobilisation, then supporting the bladder on the pelvic bone with stitches. This lessens surgical time and there's less bleeding. It also helps with stress incontinence. He only does one layer of sutures, and even then he uses very few. Just enough to hold the edges of the wound together and let them heal themselves. If there's any infection, he says, the pus will get out through the gaps.

He doesn't agree with letting patients convalesce in bed, as they do in Addis. He believes that it only produces complications, such as deep vein thrombosis. He has them up and about within a day or two of surgery.

Having whittled down his operating times, Kees can do seven or eight in a day. He hardly eats anything while he's working, just has a coffee break during the day. After finishing surgery he doesn't wait around to see how the patients are doing; he jumps in the car and drives on to the next hospital. He keeps this up for seven days a week without a day off, until his tour is finished.

Dr Biruk and Mark Bennett spent some time with Kees during one of his whirlwind trips. It was an eye-opener for both of them to see the way he works. He'd usually operate in the morning, then by about eleven o'clock he'd be in the car, hurtling at high speed over dirt roads to the next place, so as not to miss a day. Once, after a seven-hour drive, they pulled up at one of his regular hospitals and noticed a plaque that hadn't been there before. It announced that the health minister had opened a new fistula centre. It was dated the day before. Kees was furious. He'd been coming to Nigeria for 23 years, he'd cured literally thousands of women, trained many local surgeons, and they'd opened the centre without so much as a word of acknowledgment. He turned the car around and drove seven hours back again.

Biruk, like other surgeons who've watched Kees work, found some of his ideas a little too revolutionary. 'He has his own philosophy and principles. If you accept, you accept; if not, he doesn't care.'

Kees's success rate is more than 90 per cent. Andrew Browning, who puts himself somewhere between the conservative approach of Addis Ababa and the far-out techniques of Kees Waaldijk, says that his outcomes have a lot to do with his formidable skill. After 14,000 operations he's one of the most accomplished fistula surgeons in the world.

Having worked for two decades in complete obscurity Kees

was delighted that Mark and Biruk would be interested in him. 'He had tears in his eyes,' Mark remembers. 'He couldn't stop saying how happy he was that we would come and spend a week with him.'

When Mark returned to Addis, he began thinking about Kees and others like him. It seemed to him that they could help the hospital, while at the same time the hospital could help them. 'We, as an organisation, need to draw in these lone rangers as our friends and colleagues. We have a lot more resources and a longer history, but we have to change when change is necessary by what we learn from them, and we also need to encourage and support them when necessary.'

Mark suggests that helping people like Kees with equipment, or maybe even by building a new fistula centre somewhere, is a logical extension of what the Hamlins began. 'We haven't forgotten Ethiopia; we're moving ahead with our plan here, but here's a colleague who's had the same vision somewhere else and we're supporting him in what's happening there too.'

Mark proposed that they bring all of these scattered Samaritans together and form an International Society of Obstetric Fistula Surgeons. The first meeting took place in Addis Ababa in April 2007. Dr Catherine Hamlin was elected president; Dr Kees Waaldijk, vice-president; and Dr Biruk Tafesse, secretary. They resolved to get together formally once a year to exchange information and ideas.

Kees is an atheist. This bothers some of his missionary colleagues, but not Catherine. She's the first to acknowledge his accomplishments. 'He's done terribly good work, he's cured a lot of women in that area, he's written a book, he takes photos of every case and he's so enthusiastic about it.

'When he's in Nigeria he lives very spartanly, in absolute degradation. He said to Mark and Biruk, "You can't stay here, you'll have to go to a hotel." But the hotel was worse than the house.

'He was very chuffed to be asked to come. He said, "Nobody's recognised anything that I've done except you." He was so pleased.'

Dr Tom Raassen is another unsung saviour who has worked for many years in Africa. Tom is also Dutch, living in Kenya. He works with the African Medical and Research Foundation's flying doctor service, flying all over Somalia, Uganda, Rwanda, Kenya, Tanzania, southern Sudan, doing plastic surgery – things like repairing harelips and cleft palates – and fistulas.

Dr Brian Hancock spent most of his working life as a colorectal surgeon in Britain. In late 1969, early in his career, he had worked as a general surgeon at Kamuli Mission Hospital in Uganda. When he saw his first fistula cases he became fascinated by the challenge. He read the work of the British expert Professor Chassar Moir, who had written eloquently of the rewards of fistula surgery:

Nothing can equal the gratitude of the woman who, wearied by constant pain, and desperate with the realisation that her very presence is an offence to others, finds suddenly that life has been given anew, and that she has again become a citizen of the world.

Professor Moir had been helpful to the Hamlins when they were starting out. Brian also read Reg Hamlin's publications. Armed with this theoretical knowledge he did twelve fistula operations with good results.

In 1982 Brian went to Ethiopia in his holidays, where he

visited the Fistula Hospital. He was overwhelmed by what he saw there. When he went back home to England he started fund-raising. In 1988 he returned to do a locum while Reg and Catherine went on their three-yearly leave. He kept going back to do locums, and on his holidays he'd go out to do some of the difficult rectal surgeries.

Brian retired from full-time work in 2000 and started a charity called Uganda Childbirth Injuries Fund. He now spends three months of every year visiting three different hospitals in Uganda to do fistula surgery, and has also worked for Mercy Ships in several West African countries. He estimates he's done about a thousand cases. As well as developing his surgical skills, he has a passion for teaching. He's made teaching videos and has written a book called *First Steps in Fistula Surgery*. Now a second, more advanced, book is about to be published.

Dr John Kelly has been associated with the Hamlins for 38 years. He used to be the Assistant Professor of Obstetrics and Gynae-cology at Queen Elizabeth University Hospital in Birmingham, UK. In the early days at Princess Tsehai he'd visit Reg and Cath-erine to help out when they were short of doctors. He was one of the founding members of the Hamlin Churchill Childbirth Injuries Fund in Britain; he is now the chairman of the trust.

John learnt fistula surgery from the Hamlins and retired two years before he needed to, so that he could work in Africa. He travels frequently to operate on patients in Sudan, Somalia, Uganda, Tanzania, Zambia, Nigeria and Pakistan. Wars don't stop him. He has made regular visits to trouble spots in Sudan and Somalia.

Dr Jerry Putman is an American obstetrician and gynaecologist who gave up his job to work at a fistula hospital in Sierra Leone. Surgeons from Addis had been making regular trips to work on the Mercy Ship. There was such a need in Sierra Leone that in 2005 they opened a land-based hospital, the Aberdeen Clinic and Fistula Centre. Managed and operated by the Mercy Ships, it has a 44-bed ward and capacity to treat 500 to 600 patients a year.

Dr Michael Breen did his surgical training in Dublin, Ireland. He's in charge of a dedicated fistula unit at the Catholic Mission Hospital in Monze, in the south of Zambia. He originally trained in Addis Ababa and runs his hospital along similar lines, with visiting volunteer surgeons coming from the UK to perform specialised procedures.

With 90 per cent of the population earning less than two dollars a day, Zambia is one of the poorest African countries. Dr Breen estimates that there are about 500 new fistula cases every year.

Dr Steven Arrowsmith, an American urologist, saw his first fistula in 1987, when he was in his last year of residency at a hospital in Liberia. He was called to the hospital at three o'clock one morning to treat a woman with a 'humungous hole' in her bladder. Shocked by her condition, he assisted a local physician who surgically repaired her injury.

That experience touched off a lifetime interest in the problem of fistula. Dr Arrowsmith founded a fistula centre at Evangel Hospital in Jos, Nigeria, then served as Associate Medical Director at the Addis Ababa Fistula Hospital for three years. Like all fistula surgeons, he was moved by the desperate social situation of sufferers, which sometimes leads to suicide. One of the most harrowing stories he encountered was a group of West African women, despairing of their wretched condition, having chained themselves together and thrown themselves in the water to drown.

Dr Arrowsmith is the Fistula Program Coordinator for the Mercy Ships. He's also associated with the World Wide Fistula Fund, based in Illinois, USA. The fund was established in 1995 by another American surgeon, Dr Lewis Wall, to raise money for the construction of fistula centres in Africa. Dr Arrowsmith says of his colleague, 'While the faculty and staff at Washington University know Dr Wall from hospital rounds or from lecture halls, I know him from cramped bush taxis and smelly hospital wards in some of the world's poorest places.

'We have in Dr Wall a real treasure. His imposing academic credentials have given us entry into the highest levels of international policy, yet he is completely willing to work in hospitals where there is occasional electricity, and where we reuse paper surgical gowns until they fall to pieces.'

In 2003, UNFPA launched their global campaign to eradicate obstetric fistula by 2015. With an initial $20 million from a variety of donors, they have been working in partnership with NGOs in over 40 countries in Africa, Asia and the Arab region. Fistula centres have begun opening in hospitals all over the place. Many of the surgeons have been trained at Addis Ababa; others have learnt their skills from these dedicated and largely unrecognised western doctors.

The pool of fistula surgeons in Africa and Asia is growing. With the internet, doctors in isolated parts of the world are able to communicate with one another. Since the beginning of fistula surgery, various classification systems have been developed to describe the injury. James Marion Sims invented one in the mid-nineteenth century, based on site. The Hamlins developed a system, also based on site. The trouble with that is that big fistulas may spread over different sites in the vagina. If, say, it borders both the urethra and the cervix, how would you describe it? Do you call it a juxta-urethral or a juxta-cervical?

There have been many attempts to come up with a universal system. In 2002 a meeting of fistula surgeons in Geneva tried to reach an agreement. Kees Waaldijk was there, and he had what was then the most researched classification system in the world. It, too, was based on site – specifically, how much of the urethra was involved. The trouble was, it didn't include anything else.

The meeting ended without a consensus, but they did agree that the ideal system should include site, size and scarring.

Andrew Browning did some research and came up with four independent predictors for poor outcomes in fistula surgery. They were: the site of the fistula related to how much of the urethra was involved (the more involvement the worse the outcome); the size of the hole; scarring (the more scarring the worse the outcome); and size of bladder (the smaller the bladder the worse the outcome). Andrew thought this last one wasn't much help in a third-world hospital as it's difficult to measure bladder capacity before an operation unless you've got urodynamic equipment.

Judith Goh, who had done such a lot of work with fistula surgery and urinary incontinence, came up with a three-tiered system based on site, size and scarring. Site is a measurement of the number of centimetres from the edge of the fistula to the urethra. It's either a 1, a 2, a 3 or a 4. A 1 means the distance to the edge of the fistula is bigger than 3.5 centimetres. This means the sphincteric muscles are still intact, so if you can close the fistula the patient will probably be continent. A 2 is when the distance between the urethra and the edge of the fistula is 2.5 to 3.5 centimetres; 3 is 1.5 to 2.5 centimetres; 4 is less than 1.5 centimetres.

The size of the fistula will be either an A, B or C. A is 1.5 centimetres, B is 1.5 to 3 centimetres, C is bigger than 3 centimetres.

Scarring is also classified as one, two or three, written as i, ii, iii.

Andrew Browning uses Dr Goh's system, and this is the one he teaches his students. Once every two days he confers on the internet with surgeons in Asia and Africa. If a colleague tells him that he has a 4Biii, he then knows exactly what advice to offer.

Different surgeons working in different pockets of the world have all come up with slightly different systems. Biruk has developed one which is more detailed than Judith Goh's; at the time of writing it has not been studied. Some differences are: determining whether or not a patient has been operated on previously, the size of the bladder – which Biruk contends that you can measure approximately, without urodynamic equipment, by inserting a probe from the fistula to the back of the bladder, and measuring the amount of healthy tissue left, rather than the amount of scarring.

Once the International Federation of Gynaecologists and Obstetricians or the International Society of Urologists approves a classification system, it will become the international standard. Then, surgeons the world over will speak the same clinical language at last.

CHAPTER 22

Einar Lande looks like the left-wing activist he once was, back in his university days in Norway. The day I meet him in Yirgalem he's wearing creased brown slacks, with an open-neck shirt hanging out, socks and sandals. Very European. He's going bald on top and the hair that's left at the sides needs cutting. He looks as though he could do with a shave as well. He's not one of your crisply starched, shirt-and-tie doctors. But then, if he were, he probably wouldn't want to be here in an obscure corner of an impoverished African country, operating on penniless, incontinent women.

Einar's had a thing about Africa ever since he worked in Zimbabwe in the mid-1980s. He began his professional life as a general practitioner in Norway. By his mid-thirties he'd decided that he didn't like it, so he got a job in a country which is about as different from Norway as you can find – Zimbabwe. He worked in the government district hospital at Mutoko, 140 kilometres from the Zimbabwian capital, Harare.

Those years, 1985 to 1987, were the most exciting in his career to date. Zimbabwe had not yet disintegrated into the basket case that it is today. The health system worked well, he enjoyed his job, he liked his colleagues and he had a nice social life.

The doctors in Mutoko were expected to do caesarean sections, which Einar found strange, as in Norway caesareans are the strict preserve of gynaecologists. Einar had never done a caesarean in his life, and he didn't know how. 'People laughed at me. You say you're a doctor and you don't know how to do a caesarean section? They couldn't believe it.'

He spent a month in Harare learning, and by the time he'd finished, his whole outlook had changed. He decided he wanted to do two things in the future: learn gynaecology and obstetrics, and practise in an African country.

It took five years of study to fulfil the first ambition. The second took a lot longer. He set up practice, divorced, remarried and fathered two more sons to add to the one from his first marriage. Somehow the years just went by, and he still hadn't been back to Africa. But the dream remained alive. 'I still had it inside me to do meaningful work.'

One day he met a Swedish doctor who'd been in Kenya with an organisation called the Doctor Bank. They exchanged stories about working in Africa, and his new friend asked him if he'd like to come with him next time he went. 'I was thinking about the house, the bank loan and so on, and said, how is the salary? Oh no, there's no salary. I said okay. We were paid ten dollars a day, enough for food.'

Einar spent four weeks at a little hospital at Garissa, near the Somali border. One of his patients was a woman who arrived on the bus already in labour. She'd been trying to deliver for four days. Einar did a caesarean and delivered a stillborn baby. It was his first encounter with the cruel realities of women's medicine in a developing country, and the first time he'd seen a fistula. 'I wanted to call for my mother, because all was ruptured and torn. I hadn't seen that working with obstetrics in Norway.'

The next day Tom Raassen arrived on one of his flying visits. Einar asked if he would teach him how to repair fistulas. Tom refused, telling him that he didn't train doctors who lived and worked in Europe.

Einar could have gone home and taken up where he left off, living a comfortable life, working in his practice, enjoying walks in the forest with his friends, but he could not get that woman out of his mind. He got in touch with the Addis Ababa Fistula Hospital and asked if he could train there. They refused. Like Tom, they were concerned that he was just another fistula tourist. When a further trip to Garissa came up, Einar asked again if he could come to Addis on his way there, just as an observer, to see what went on. They relented.

That was in 2002. Einar watched the doctors at work, but without hands-on experience he didn't learn a great deal. 'It was very difficult to get into the world of fistulas. I wanted that, and I had a wife who was prepared to go along with it, but it was very difficult. It was like everyone was pushing me away.'

Another three years went by. A Norwegian church organisation asked if he'd work for three months in the Congo where they had a fistula program. He said he was interested, and he'd like to do it but had not actually done any fistula surgery. Also, he didn't speak French.

They told him that none of that was a problem. While he was keen to go, Einar thought his inexperience most likely *was* a problem. He contacted the Fistula Hospital once more. After hearing that he was going to work in the Congo, their attitude was quite different. They agreed to give him ten days of training, which was all that he had time for. Feeling a little more confident, he then went to Bukavu near the Rwandan border, where there had been a lot of war and rape and murder going on.

The program was for women who had sustained their fistulas

as a result of gang rape, or being assaulted with blunt instruments. He was told by the head of the program that 75 per cent of their patients had been raped. During his three months there he saw 150 patients and asked each one of them how they had got their fistula. Every one had been after childbirth. 'Personally I didn't like this. It's bad enough to have a fistula, let alone having to lie and say it was because of rape. So they made the project a little bit dishonest.' Einar kept his mouth shut about his misgivings, on the basis that any program that gave money for fistula patients had to be a good thing.

One of his colleagues in the Congo was a self-taught fistula surgeon. He told Einar that he'd give him the simple cases and he'd train him. He ended up doing about 40.

Even after that experience it was difficult to find the work he wanted, until a Norwegian friend, Professor Torvid Kiserud, from Bergen University, told him he was about to visit Addis Ababa. Torvid is a professor of obstetrics and gynaecology. His university had formed an alliance with Addis to help them with research. In the past the Ethiopian doctors had had trouble publishing papers because of the difficulty of mastering the specific style of language required. One of Torvid's tasks was to help them in this area.

Einar asked his friend to enquire about a job for him. Yirgalem was soon to open, and in early 2006 he received a text message with the news he had been hoping for. 'I was very happy. It was all impossible economically and all the rest of it, but I told my wife if I don't do this I'll regret it the rest of my life.'

We're sitting in the lounge room of Einar's house. The plumbing is forever giving trouble; his cook doesn't know how to make anything that he likes, so he does most of the cooking himself; his nearest European neighbours are at Awassa, 40 kilometres away; his wife and two of his sons are in Norway. One good thing is that his ten-year-old, Johnathan, is living with him and Einar's enjoying having lots of time with him.

Johnathan is the sort of kid who's up for anything new. He told his dad that he was prepared to come to Ethiopia for five or six years. He's being educated at Awassa, in a little school for the children of Danish missionaries. There are only four students. Johnathan travels to Awassa with the hospital driver and spends a couple of nights during the week with a schoolfriend's parents.

In Norway, Johnathan's teachers used to tell Einar that his son had learning difficulties. Something's changed. 'Here all of a sudden he's normal. They say, "We don't see any learning difficulties." It makes me so happy I start crying. It's nice for me that he's so happy. In Norway we only had meetings about my son being a problem.'

Johnathan's enjoying Ethiopia. Einar's thirteen-year-old, Mattis, on the other hand, isn't keen on the idea of living there. Einar's asked him to give it a try for six months. Soon he's going to rent a house in Addis, then Mattis and his mother, Catherine, will come out. Mattis can go to one of the foreign schools in Addis, and Catherine will probably find work as a teacher. Einar's got a contract for a year. He's been in Ethiopia five months already. He's promised his family that if they don't like it after spending six months here, he'll go back home. Meanwhile he's getting on with the job of running the hospital, being paid the same salary as the Ethiopian surgeons. He thinks this is fine. It doesn't cost a lot to live the way he does.

With no other Europeans around, it's a quiet and lonely life. At home he'd be out walking or running in the forest three or four times a week. 'I miss that. But movies, restaurants and so on, I don't miss. The work is so inspiring for me, much more than what I do at home. So if it's possible for me to do this for many years I would, but I don't know, because I must keep all my promises to my son. If he says "I want to go home", I'll go home.'

I ask Einar the same question I ask every fistula surgeon I meet. Why? He says, 'I think maybe it's a bit arrogant, but technically most of the time it's not that difficult, but it's this feeling that what I do has a meaning.'

While he's talking he's opening up his laptop computer. The screen illuminates and he turns it towards me. 'I want to show you a smile. I sent this to a midwife friend and asked her, "Do you understand what I'm talking about?"'

There's a picture of a beautiful girl in her teens, sitting on a bed. She's looking straight at the camera with an expression of pure bliss. It speaks to me as if she were here in the room.

'That's the first patient I operated on,' says Einar. 'You don't have to ask if she was cured.'

The pathways to this profession are varied. Many fistula surgeons do it because of their Christian faith. There's a plaque in the hospital at Addis Ababa commemorating Reg Hamlin's life of service. It includes a quote from Jesus, as written in the gospel of Matthew: 'Whoever helps the least of these my brothers, helps me.' Reg and Catherine Hamlin certainly believed that. But what about these lone rangers like Kees Waaldijk? Or Einar Lande?

It's not faith that drives Einar. He's a lukewarm Christian at best. He doesn't go to church and he's uncomfortable about the motives of a lot of missionaries. 'Once I tried to get a job through the Norwegian Lutheran mission,' he tells me. 'They asked what I thought of missionaries. I said I'm sceptical, because it's a way of buying people. A good missionary friend said the reason you have trouble getting a job in Africa is because your relationship to religion is not strong enough. But I cannot fake it. Not that

I don't believe. I've been a bit upset about that, because I want to do a job.'

The general hospital in Yirgalem to which the fistula centre is attached was built by a Norwegian mission. They've now handed it over to the government to run. Einar thinks it's wrong to use medicine to spread the gospel and then leave. 'I feel that missionaries should stay forever, like Mrs Hamlin. For me she is an example of a good Christian missionary. I've heard in some countries patients are ill in hospital and missionaries come and want to christen them. That's not a fair situation. I've heard of people saying yes, just so they can get the treatment. I don't think Mrs Hamlin and her husband did that. I admire that woman a lot. She's really a good, Christian person, and she's treating people very nicely without pushing her faith onto them.'

Einar has fallen under Catherine's spell, as everyone does. It's the little kindnesses that impress him. When he was travelling down from Addis to take up his post, he had a little dog in the car. Catherine bought a basket for it to sleep in and gave him a sheet, in case the dog got carsick. 'It threw up three times, Einar remembers. 'That sheet saved me.'

She wrote him a note wishing him well in his new job. When he read it he said to himself, 'I think I love her already.'

Einar leans towards the Andrew Browning school. His patients get out of bed a day or so after surgery and walk around carrying their little buckets. His rounds are freewheeling affairs. He jokes a lot with the nurses, and nurse aides; sometimes even asks their opinion about what to do. He doesn't try to hide his doubts about his ability to handle difficult cases. He tries hard to be nice to everyone, from the matron all the way down to the cooks. I get the feeling that this approach is a bit mystifying to his staff, who are used to a strict hierarchy.

There are 25 beds in the ward, but many of them are empty. As with the other new centres, the patients have been slow to come. They're getting about one a day. There's a woman waiting patiently on a bench at outpatients – a typical rural woman, with travel-stained clothing and a few possessions at her feet in a plastic bag. Einar excuses himself and takes her into the examination room.

After about twenty minutes he comes out and directs her to the hospital next door. He looks downhearted. She was suffering from incontinence, but he's discovered that it wasn't due to a fistula. She has cancer of the cervix. He thinks it's inoperable, but wants the gynaecologist at the government hospital to give a second opinion.

'When I saw this I felt like leaving the room,' he says. 'It upsets me.'

In Norway she would have radiation, which would prolong her life. The Black Lion in Addis does it but she'd have to pay and wait in the queue. They don't prioritise. Even hopeless cases go before ones of people who could be saved.

He hasn't told her that she has cancer. He's worried about how it would come out in translation. And he wants that other opinion first. 'I just told her that she's seriously ill and I don't know if she can be cured.'

Einar wants to know why patients aren't coming to him. One day we set off in the hospital Toyota to drive to Hagere Selam, the administrative centre of this *woreda*, or district. With us are one of the nurses and the gateman. We need two people to translate, one from the local language, Sidama, into Amharic, the other from Amharic to English.

The road winds up and down emerald-green hillsides,

splashed with banana plantations and fields of *chat*. *Chat* leaves contain cathinone, an amphetamine-like stimulant. Chewing them induces mild euphoria and a feeling of wellbeing. Since the coffee price collapsed many farmers have changed over to growing *chat*. You see bunches of it on sale everywhere. It's addictive. People lose their will to work and instead sit around idly, chewing the stuff all day. In extreme cases it can cause psychosis. *Chat* has become a blight on Ethiopian society.

Nestled into the greenery are clusters of round *tukuls*. It's rich country, this. The views from the hilltops are breathtaking. But you know that hidden away in those picture-postcard settlements are women living lives of misery.

People stroll nonchalantly down the middle of the road. They drift out from the side without looking and then appear surprised to see a car almost on top of them. There are donkeys carrying loads, herds of goats, the occasional horse-drawn cart. Hardly any motor vehicles. These roads are for people and animals, not cars.

We're climbing higher as we go, and the air is cooling. One and a quarter hours after leaving Yirgalem, we come to the top of a ridge and park in front of a health centre. It's a collection of neglected-looking buildings which were once painted yellow. The paint has mostly worn away and you can see rust-stained concrete showing through. We get out and a small group of people gathers curiously around us. They're swathed in *gabis* and jumpers and headscarves. It's cold up here. A young woman dressed in western clothing, who looks to be in her early twenties, comes out to see what the fuss is about. She says there is no doctor here but she's the midwife – the only midwife for the entire *woreda* of 120,000 people. She'll be happy to talk to us.

In reasonably good English she politely ushers us into a cramped little room. It's a bare concrete cell containing a couple of filing cabinets, a desk and an examination couch with the stuffing falling out. Through another door I can see an operating table with stirrups, also leaking stuffing. There's not a lick of paint anywhere and the floor looks as though it has never been swept. The midwife informs us that this is where she delivers babies.

Our room is crammed with women who have come for a three-monthly contraceptive injection. There's a strong smell of sweat and woodsmoke. One by one they approach the desk, fish out a battered card from the depths of their clothing and hand it over to a male nurse aide wearing a soiled blue coat. He marks the card and breaks the seal on a new syringe. They look away and he jabs them in the arm. It seems to be a joyless business on both sides. Not a word is exchanged.

Einar quizzes the midwife, and a nurse who has joined us, about the system of prenatal and postnatal care. The midwife says she does 150 deliveries a year and she has never seen a fistula. Only 150 deliveries in a *woreda* of 120,000. It's a mystery why she doesn't do more. Or maybe not such a mystery, when you look at these facilities.

Einar questions her for a long time. He's very thorough. He wants to be sure that he understands everything correctly. When he's finished she takes us on a tour. She shows us into another little concrete room with two mattresses on the floor. Two women with infants are sitting on the mattresses. She explains that they're here because their children have been suffering from poor nutrition. The floor is littered with trash, a few empty feeding bottles are mixed up with the mess. It's freezing cold and everything is dirty. It's hard to imagine that the children's health will improve here.

Hagere Selam is just a few minutes' drive away. It's a small town, in the centre of which is a wide, wind-blown square. It's crammed full of men wandering aimlessly about. There's not a woman in sight. I wonder where they all are? Our car noses through the crowd like a predator through a school of fish. People peel aside and stare in through the windows as we pass. Our gateman asks for directions to the administrative centre and we inch our way across the square and up a steep dirt road pockmarked with foot-deep potholes.

The administrative centre is a distempered building behind a falling-down corrugated-iron fence. At the end of a long, dark and very dirty corridor is the office of the director of health. The director is away but his second-in-charge is there. He graciously welcomes us.

Einar tells him that he's from the new fistula hospital which has opened in Yirgalem. The assistant director's never heard of it. He knows about the one in Addis but this most recent one is news to him.

On the wall behind the assistant director's desk are some statistical charts. The total population of Hula Woreda, the district we are in, is 121,481. There are 59,526 females and an estimated 5175 births per year. The World Health Organization calculates that there are three fistulas for every thousand births. By that reckoning they should be seeing at least fifteen a year.

'We never see any,' he says.

'Why not?'

'Because hardly anyone has their child in a medical facility. Yirgalem is the closest place they can go for a caesarean, and they would have to catch a bus or hire a vehicle to get there.'

The assistant director is keen to help. He says he'll ask his extension workers to go house to house and enquire about fistula sufferers. And also inform people that there's a fistula hospital in Yirgalem. 'But it could be that they are ashamed and hiding,' he warns.

The southern region of Ethiopia, which is the Yirgalem fistula hospital's catchment area, has a population of 17 million people. There must be thousands of sufferers out there, yet the new hospital has only seen 150 cases.

Einar takes heart from the experience at Bahar Dar. Hopefully, it will only be a matter of time before he, too, has as much work as he can handle.

CHAPTER 23

When I return to Addis Ababa from Yirgalem I run into Amina in the garden. She gives me a big smile and seizes both my hands and kisses them. She gestures at the ground. It's dry. This is great news. I wish I could talk to her or give her a hug, but neither of these things is possible. So I just say an enthusiastic 'Okay', and give her the thumbs up. She understands.

The nursing sister in charge of the Bethlehem ward, Sister Hannah, tells me that Amina has been going to Sister Azeb for pelvic floor exercises. She's not completely continent but is a lot better than she was. She's just about ready to go home. They'll advise her to wait six months and if she's still having trouble she can come back and they'll try an operation.

I expect Catherine to be pleased when I see her, but she has some news which immediately squashes my enthusiasm. She has learnt that Amina has not had any periods since she gave birth. They're sometimes late restarting after childbirth, but not usually this late. Catherine suspects it's another case of the surgeon who did the caesarean removing her uterus without telling her.

This is terrible news. I know Amina has told me she doesn't

want to marry again, but nearly all fistula patients say that at first. She has no education and no chance of finding skilled work. Her best chance for a happy life would be to find a good man to care for her and give her children. I fear that this lovely young woman has had her life destroyed.

For the moment Catherine hasn't said anything to her. She's ordered an ultrasound which will tell if her suspicions are correct.

I've grown fond of Amina. I've been riding the rollercoaster with her. But I can get off whenever I want, and go back to my privileged existence in Australia. There's nothing she can do to change her fate. Ethiopia – Africa – is full of tragic stories. I've heard dozens of them. The difference with Amina is that I've lived the story with her. I feel as involved as if she were a member of my own family. And there's absolutely nothing I can do to change things.

At least there's good news about Zemebech. She's cured and ready to go home. 'I am very happy,' she says. 'I was crying before coming here. I was begging everyone to take me here. I knew if I had a chance to come I was sure to be cured.'

But there's a problem. Her husband left her here and went back to the village to look after their three children. One of his relatives, who lives in Addis, was meant to come back and accompany her on the trip home. Her village is far away from the nearest town and she wouldn't feel secure having to make the journey alone. The problem is that the relative hadn't planned to return until the end of the rainy season, which is three months away.

Sister Konjit says they'll try to find him. They won't just turn her out on her own.

★

Halema is also getting ready to leave. She has a phone number for her sister, who's staying with Somali friends in Addis. Biruk says her fistula is cured. When she stands up after going to the toilet there are sometimes a few drops, but that will clear up naturally. It's an amazing outcome, considering Biruk's pessimism during surgery.

Today there's a nurse aide here who can speak Somali. Through her, Halema tells me how happy she is that she's cured. 'Thanks to Allah.'

Alganish had her operation later than the others. Last time I saw her, things were not looking hopeful. She was leaking around the catheter and there was some sloughing of the wound. Catherine was worried that it might break down and have to be done again.

Alganish is in the Princess Anne ward, so named because Her Royal Highness opened it during a visit to Ethiopia. She's lying on her back asleep, with her face covered by her shawl. I don't wish to wake her. As I turn to leave she stirs, takes the shawl away, opens her eyes and stretches luxuriously. She sees me and her face lights up with her trademark smile.

Alganish is still not completely continent. She needs to stay a while yet. She's worried that her kids won't have enough to eat. She's sure their stepfather won't be looking after them while she's away. If they were able to be with their father she wouldn't be concerned.

She's philosophical about her condition. 'I have good hope for the future,' she says. 'Thanks to God I am better than when I came.'

★

I come across Leteabazgi sitting with some other girls on the patio in front of the Bethlehem ward. It's the first time I've seen her without something covering her head. Her hair is shaven up both sides and left long at the back. There's a sort of Mohican cut in the middle and a single long plait going across her forehead. I've never seen a hairstyle like it.

The last time I saw Leteabazgi she was dry, drinking and draining. From her demeanour now, something has changed. When I ask her how she is, she starts to cry. She pours out a tale of woe. The doctors have told her the fistula is cured, but she's still wet; she's been trying to do pelvic floor exercises but they're too hard; they've said she'll have to go home and come back after six months if things don't improve; she had to borrow money to get here and she's worried that she won't have enough for the bus fare; and she's afraid to travel alone.

Poor Leteabazgi. She's been up and down during the weeks that I've known her. She's way down now, reverting to the same introverted state as when she first arrived. She goes through her litany in a tiny little voice that I can barely hear, with her eyes fixed at a spot on the ground. The fistula has been closed but as far as she's concerned she's not cured.

I tell her not to worry about money. The hospital will give her some. She brightens up a bit at that. She doesn't seem to have the fortitude that most of the other patients have. I wonder if she'll be courageous enough to come back again if she has to.

So, out of six patients chosen at random, three – Letelibanes, Zemebech and Halema – have been completely cured. Amina is both better and maybe worse off than when she came. Her two fistulas have been repaired but she's still not completely continent. And soon Catherine may have to tell her that even if she does improve, she will never be a mother.

As for Alganish and Leteabazgi, we'll have to wait a little longer.

CHAPTER 24

It hardly needs saying by now that the Addis Ababa Fistula Hospital is a very special place, for both patients and staff. Some of the key people have been there for decades and intend to stay until retirement age or beyond. Matron Edjigayehu is in her mid-fifties. She radiates an aura of motherly calm, whether she's dealing with a medical emergency or a delicate personal problem with one of the nurses. She first went to the Princess Tsehai Hospital in 1965 as a student nurse. Students were assigned for one month to the outpatients clinic. Reg took a shine to her. He loved keen young people who could quickly pick up on his ideas and who could interpret for him. He nicknamed her 'Edjiy' and used his influence with the Ministry of Health so that she ended up staying for nine months.

Reg had always been a gifted teacher. Back in the days when he was the medical superintendent of Crown Street Women's Hospital in Sydney, the students all adored him. He was good at making up little ditties that helped people learn. When he lectured on abnormal deliveries, he used to say, 'If there's a problem, it's either the passage or the passenger.' They used chloroform as an anaesthetic then, and there was always a risk of overdosing the patient. You had to drip carefully only a few drops onto their mask. Reg would say, 'Always use care, prayer and plenty of air.'

At the Princess Tsehai Hospital he'd use his piece of paper to explain fistulas to the arriving patients. Then he'd go through a little pantomime for them, to show what would happen when they returned to their village after being cured. Shading his eyes, he would pretend to be one of the villagers spying a girl coming along the path. 'Who is this looking so pretty and happy? No, it can't be Hirut who went away only a few weeks ago, so wretched and sad. Why it is her, but how changed she is!' Then he would describe her reunion with her family just as vividly.

This endeared him to the patients, and it endeared him to sensitive young nurses such as Edjigayehu, who was blessed with more than the usual degree of compassion for the patients. 'Reg was very special. He loved people. He loved specially the fistula patients. There were first-class patients attending the clinic and they usually wanted Catherine. Reg liked the poor people. He hugged them and kissed them. They were special to him.'

Edjigayehu always wanted to stay with the Hamlins. But after she graduated, the Ministry of Health assigned her to other hospitals. It wasn't until 1991 that she joined the Fistula Hospital as a night nurse. She loved working with poor people. It was the patients' stories, as much as the medical side of her job, that attracted her. 'It's special every time. You hear someone's history one day and it touches your heart. Then the next day you hear another history and it's always new. It's never ever boring.'

Edjigayehu is six years off retirement. As she reflects on her time at the hospital and the startling changes that she's seen, she says, 'I am a very lucky nurse.'

★

Genet Kifle, the financial controller, has been at the hospital for twenty years. Retirement age is 65 but she says that as long as she's useful she'll stay. 'I love this place.'

She can remember when the hospital staff was like a family. Her job was to do the accounts, but often when she came in to work Reg would ask her to help out in outpatients, interpreting and admitting new patients. When she saw how he treated the smelly, wretched women who had come seeking help, she realised his humanity. 'Reg used to hug them and I was very much impressed by that. Catherine is the same. She loves the patients.'

Genet has three children. Two years after she started at the hospital she was pregnant with twins. Late in her pregnancy she arrived at work one morning and bumped into Catherine. 'How are you today?' she asked. 'Any sign of labour?'

'I think so,' said Genet.

'Come and we'll see.'

Catherine took her into outpatients, examined her and told her she was not to move. The twins were born at the Black Lion later that day. Then the Hamlins brought them back to the Fistula Hospital. 'The babies are small,' Reg told her. 'They need care.' Genet and the babies stayed for a fortnight.

Back then Genet was the only person in the office. In her lunch hour she used to visit patients just to chat and hear their stories, but the place has become too big and her workload too heavy for her to do that now.

She has three accountants working under her and they're about to hire another three to cope with the extra work from the new hospitals. They've also got a sophisticated, computerised financial management program. When Reg first hired Genet, he showed her the accounting book and told her not to worry, that they had 500,000 birr in the savings account. Now they've got about $40,000. That wouldn't go far these days: the hospital costs several million dollars a year to run, all of it raised through charity. One thing hasn't changed. Now, as then, the auditors always find that Genet's accounting is impeccable.

Zewditu Hailu is another quiet achiever, toiling away quietly out of the spotlight. She worked for a foreign-run training centre who sent her to Sweden to learn how to teach crafts. When the centre closed she spent a couple of years at home, and then Catherine approached her to teach at Desta Mender. She spent two years there, then came over to set up a crafts program at the main hospital.

Zewditu works in a little room with a small verandah in front of it which has been built behind the Bete Mesgana. It was donated by the family of an Ethiopian girl, Woubale Zewdie, who died of cancer. They decided to build something for living people rather than a marble tomb. Anyone who wants to can come along and learn embroidery, sewing, knitting, cane work and so on.

Zewditu's assistant, Hagere Getu, teaches knitting. Hagere has been at the Fistula Hospital for seven years, living in the same house up the hill where Bossena and Fatuma, the two inseparable nurse aides, live. Her parents arranged her marriage when she was twelve. She didn't like her husband, so she ran away to Addis Ababa where she met another man and started living with him.

When she became pregnant she said she wanted to go back to Gonder to be with her parents while she had the baby. She was afraid to be in Addis without their support. Her husband begged her not to go, but her mind was made up. What happened next is a familiar scenario – a long labour, a dead baby and a severely injured mother. Her husband wanted to be with her and support her, but she told him she didn't want him around anymore. This is not uncommon. Mamitu did the same thing when she was injured. Some women feel that they are no longer worthy. They are so ashamed of their condition that they tell their husbands to leave.

Hagere's injuries were so severe that she had to have a urinary diversion. Gordon Williams did a Mainz II pouch operation. The operation was successful, but Hagere slid into deep, deep depression. She remained curled up in bed all day, refusing to look at anyone or to respond to questions. Her eyes were glazed and she had a blank look. She was in a psychotic state.

They gave her anti-depressant drugs and counselled her, and one day she started knitting a cardigan. Something about that activity brought her back to life. When she finished the cardigan she asked if she could have some more wool. She finished a second cardigan and went on to a third. After months of being removed from the world, suddenly she was knitting constantly. It had changed her completely.

Ruth suggested to Matron that they ask Hagere if she'd like to teach knitting. They gave her a uniform, and now she teaches girls to knit, and she braids unusual and very artistic mats and cushion covers, using the legs of the stockings that Gordon brings. She sells them to visitors for 10 birr.

Hagere is 30. She has a tattooed jawline and wears her hair in tight little cornrows. She wears spectacles – these and a perpetually serious look on her face give her a studious air.

Every day up to a dozen patients come to learn a whole range of crafts. I've been listening to patients' stories for weeks, but still they amaze me. There's Abebech, sitting quietly embroidering a tablecloth with a pretty design of flowers. Married at ten, got her fistula with her second child, 40 years old now and waiting for an operation. She should have come here a long time ago, but her father died and her mother is blind, so she had to take care of her brothers and sisters until they were old enough to leave home. Her husband is a priest. He was furious with her when she was injured. He can't divorce her but he no longer lives with her. He spends all his time in church praying.

Next to her, there's a beautiful girl, Yirgalem, from Shoa. She's eighteen, married at fourteen. She's had a colostomy. Now she's waiting for the operation to repair her fistula and then she'll have another to restore the diversion.

Abeba is from Afar. She's 21. Both her parents are dead. Her husband deserted her, so she's got no one to look after her. She's waiting for an operation. Sometimes she sells something she's made, to visitors. With the money she earns she's saving up to buy a pair of shoes or some oil for her hair.

Yitaesh is 46, from Gojjam. She's had twelve children; seven died. It was having twins that gave her a fistula. She had three operations and she's still not cured, so she's waiting to have a fourth.

Asafu is from Wollo. She's heavily tattooed on her forehead, nose and chin. She thinks she's about 24. She's laughing merrily with her friends at the *ferenji* asking all these questions. When I ask her for her story she suddenly becomes serious. She's had her fistula for ten years, she says, so if she is 24 it must have happened when she was fourteen.

Why has it taken so long to come here? Because the hospital she went to just gave her different medicines. They didn't know what the problem was. If I'd heard this story three weeks ago I wouldn't have believed it. How could trained medical professionals not recognise a fistula when they are so common? But having heard so many other hospital horror stories I'm ready to believe that it's true.

Asafu has had her fistula closed but she has stress incontinence. She has to wait three months for another operation. I'm amazed at her cheeriness. She's always smiling, says Zewditu.

There are half a dozen others, all sitting happily sewing and embroidering and knitting, bonded by the ordeals they've shared. Zewditu's heard dozens of these stories, and every time she hears one she feels sad. 'But what can we do?' she says. 'It's our country's problem. If we get better hospitals and doctors it will be better.' Although she doesn't like to question her students, after a while their stories always come out. 'They like to talk. Mostly they miss their parents. Without them they feel like a child. Also, their husbands don't treat them well. But that's life.'

When Zewditu started the craft program it was hard to get people to come. Many were too shy or traumatised. So she did something that every Ethiopian could relate to – she began having a coffee ceremony every afternoon after lunch. Anyone who wants to come just turns up. The students take it in turns to make the coffee and serve it in the tiny cups. Zewditu always has little treats, such as boiled corn kernels or maize, to pass around. It's such a friendly little gathering that attendance has spread beyond her students. Nurse aides, admin staff, cleaners, teachers, and even some of the men turn up. They sit around, sip their coffee, chat, joke a bit. There's laughter now and then and even Hagere sometimes manages a smile. A little bit of normality. And, Lord knows, they need it.

CHAPTER 25

One morning at a prayer breakfast in Addis Ababa, Ruth found herself sitting next to the World Bank's representative in Ethiopia, John Riverson. As they munched their toast, Mr Riverson told her with pride what the World Bank was doing about HIV/AIDS. When he'd finished, Ruth said, 'That's great, but what are you doing about maternal health?'

'What is there to do?'

'Plenty.'

Never one to let an opportunity pass, Ruth gave him a rundown on the problem of obstetric fistula. She told him how women found it impossible to get to hospital because there were no roads, how women couldn't reach care because trucks wouldn't pick them up, how women in the rainy season couldn't even get from their village to the nearest basic health facility because the roads were blocked with torrents of water.

'Write a paper about it,' said Mr Riverson, which Ruth did. He attached it to his report and sent it off to Washington.

That was ten years ago. The World Bank works slowly, but in this case it did work. A couple of years later Dr Mulu was invited to speak in Addis at a workshop on maternal health, where she mentioned many of the same things Ruth had brought up. Among the visitors were representatives of the Japanese government. Everyone went away and wrote their reports and nothing happened for three or four years. Then the hospital was surprised to learn that the Japanese government was offering $2 million to the World Bank for the development of all-weather trailways and bridges, and providing access to transport for rural women to get to health facilities. The idea was to supply women with easily recognisable laminated cards, which they could hold out so that trucks would stop and give them a lift.

More time passed, until, about a year ago, the Fistula Hospital was invited to manage the project. Ruth and Mulu told the World Bank that they didn't have the skills; their business was repairing fistulas. They suggested it should be managed by the Ethiopian Road Authority. The ERA said they'd be willing and took it to the Ministry of Health. The ministry told them if the Fistula Hospital wouldn't manage it they didn't want the project. The trustees discussed it, and rather than let the project fall through they agreed that they'd handle it, thinking that perhaps they could outsource the work. Then suddenly the Ministry of Health was back in the picture, saying that *they* would have to handle it. So round and round they go. Maybe one day it will happen.

Without doubt a network of trailways would make a difference to maternal health and help reduce the number of fistulas. But even if women in labour can find their way to a health facility in time, the resources are pitifully poor.

There are only 1189 midwives in all Ethiopia for a population of 78 million people. Eighty-five per cent of people live in a rural setting, yet the majority of health professionals are based in the cities. Ninety-five per cent of women give birth without professional assistance. That's the main reason why, despite all the thousands of fistulas they've been repairing in Addis and the outreach hospitals, the number is still increasing.

Reg and Catherine Hamlin originally came to Ethiopia to set up a school of midwifery. In 1959, as now, there were pitifully few midwives in the country. Reg got in touch with a famous tutor-midwife, Miss Maggie Myles of Scotland. Miss Myles was the author of the best textbook on the subject at the time. She agreed to come to Addis Ababa to help get the school under way; the first students were honoured to have the best teacher in the world.

Miss Myles set up the curriculum, did some teaching and worked with the tutor-sister in the government nursing school at Princess Tsehai Hospital. She donated many of her own textbooks to the library.

With this excellent tuition the first midwives graduated and all of them went on to teaching jobs themselves. Reg and Catherine were pleased to have made such a good beginning, but that was as far as it went. The Ministry of Health decided it would be too expensive to pay nurses the extra money for being midwives. They saw no reason why ordinary nurses couldn't look after women in labour.

Catherine has been telling the government for decades that the way to solve the problem of obstetric fistula, as well as many other maternal health problems, is by having a proper network of trained midwives. The message just doesn't seem to get through.

When Ruth Kennedy worked for the Ministry of Health she got an insight into how the best-intentioned initiatives can be strangled by the bureaucracy. She and another midwife set up an organisation called Midwifery Updating Skills Training (MUST). The aim was to go to different hospitals, work in the labour and delivery room for a week doing cleaning and practical work, and then for a second week, train the nurses in emergency obstetrics. 'We presented the proposal and were told, "Yes, this is nice". We were then given the runaround. It took six months to release $5000 for us to do this. When we got the $5000 we started going places. We bought rubber gloves, soap powder and cleaning supplies and started visiting every region. Between 1998 and '99 we'd visit the hospitals, put on our uniforms and gloves and for one week we'd clean and we'd wash. We paid for painters to come in and paint. We wrote reports, and sent them to the minister and to UNFPA who funded us. To this day they're the only reports they have on the condition of maternal health services.'

About five years ago the government implemented a plan to train 30,000 health extension workers. They took tenth-grade graduates and gave them a year's training, including basic instruction about deliveries. It has done nothing to lower the rate of complications with childbirth. As I write this, plans are in place to improve outcomes by giving them a further two months' training.

Dr Mulu has grave reservations about this initiative. 'Obstetrics isn't as narrow as that. Maybe this two months' training might help them to identify obstructed labour and refer them, but they won't be able to do the deliveries themselves. I feel that it's a waste of money. You'll see maybe in two years or so, after training 30,000 people and wasting all those resources, the government may say there's no difference in death and disability, so let's try something else.'

Mulu repeats what Catherine and every other fistula surgeon knows. Death and injury due to childbirth can only be reduced through the attendance of a skilled birth attendant, and this, at a minimum, has to be a midwife.

'Rather than training 30,000 health extension workers,' Mulu adds, 'I would have preferred to use that money to train 5000 midwives, and then place them in 5000 villages in central areas.'

Catherine had often thought about founding her own school of midwifery, but there were never the resources to do it. When money began pouring in three or four years ago, at last it seemed like a possibility. Not everyone thought it was a good idea. The American trust was against it, on the grounds that it was not related directly to fistula. Charities have to be very careful about going off on tangents that don't fit in with their charter.

Mark Bennett went to the US and argued that a midwifery school would be very much part of preventing fistula. The trustees listened and changed their minds. By 2006 Catherine, Ruth, Mark, and his wife, Annette, had drawn up a plan and a budget. It has been serendipitous that Annette is a midwife. There was also a trained male midwife on staff, Solomon Abebe, who had been helping to set up the new regional centres. In early 2007 Annette and Solomon were joined in Addis Ababa by the Professor of Midwifery at Manchester University in England, Ann Thomson, and they began drawing up a curriculum.

Catherine's plan is to choose students not from the provincial capitals but from rural areas. 'It's very important to select girls who we think will go back and stay in their own area. Then we'll have a birthing centre for them, possibly near a health centre. And we say, "We're coming to see you every few months to see how you're getting on". Don't leave them out on a limb, give them all the equipment they need, pay them a decent salary, build them a little house to live in and then they would soon get to know all the women in the district, even villages a bit further away from their own village. They'll get to know them and visit them and become part of their family. Then they'll get the trust of these people.

'The main thing is not to leave them feeling deserted when they're in these little centres. We're going to put two in each so they'll have a companion. Also, they might be overwhelmed with work, and you can't be up day and night delivering women.'

Listening to Catherine outlining her vision is like listening to an enthusiastic new recruit. The ideas tumble out in a torrent. There will eventually be 25 midwifery centres. It will cost $3500 to train a midwife, $25,000 a year to run a clinic. That's a total cost of about $1 million a year for 25 clinics. She plans to build the first centres within 50 kilometres of the new fistula hospitals, so that there will be somewhere to refer obstructed labours. 'We want them to be able to pick out the women who they think might need a caesarean section. A good midwife can do that on the lie of the baby inside the mother – if it's abnormal, or if they're very short, if the head's not fitting in properly in the last month of pregnancy – the head should be engaged in the pelvis, not wobbling about above the brim. You can palpate and feel it.

'My husband's written a very good book on midwifery. It describes all those manoeuvres that we used to do. All the old obstetricians were very good at turning babies round and so on. This is what we have to be able to do. The old-fashioned midwifery is so important here. We've got some old midwives, then this professor with all her modern techniques. We'll have a vehicle that can go out. We'll say to the health worker, "If you can get the woman to the main road we'll get the car." We'll get mobile phones for them all so they can contact the centres.'

Annette, Ann and Solomon have spent weeks devising the curriculum. It will have to be approved by the Ministry of Education, which may well turn out to be difficult. Under the Ethiopian curriculum, students do a lot of rote learning. When they graduate they are able to regurgitate large volumes of information, but are very short on practical experience. Some graduates have gone on immediately to tutoring, after having only done six deliveries.

The team wants to encourage the development of problem-solving skills and practical initiative, rather than rote learning. This will be a radical shift away from what the students are used to right from their earliest learning experience. They will have to teach the students a new way to learn.

No one is sure what the ministry will think of this. Catherine and Ruth are preparing themselves for a fight if need be. They're old hands at dealing with government ministers. They never make an appointment, the two of them just turn up. Ruth says jokingly that Catherine is her *laisser passer* (free pass), because she's been here so long and everyone knows her.

'That's all I'm good for now,' retorts Catherine, with a chuckle.

'When we get in we just bulldoze our way through,' says Ruth. 'I'm not above a bit of blackmail, either, if need be. If there's a problem I'll say, "Oh dear, I wonder what the President will think when I have to tell him we can't start the midwives school?"'

I can just see Ruth doing it. Once, when she was in Chad, she went to the Chief of Police to get approval for an exit visa. The chief, who had taken over the job after killing his predecessor, was sitting in a darkened office wearing sunglasses and had a gun on his desk.

'This passport isn't in order,' he said.

'Oh, really? I used it to leave the country just a month ago.'

'No, it's not in order and you're in trouble. I'm going to put you in jail.'

Ruth quietly prayed while he shuffled the pages. Suddenly he stopped and looked up. 'Your name is Kennedy?'

'Yes.'

'Your father is John Kennedy?'

'Yes, that's right.'

'Maybe we can give you a visa after all.'

At the airport when she left, everyone's luggage was spread out on the tarmac being searched. Ruth's luggage was untouched. She sailed straight through Immigration without so much as a question.

We're in the hospital Toyota on the way to church when she tells this story. 'I never told a lie,' she insists. 'My father's name is John Kennedy. If he chose to believe he was the American president it wasn't up to me to tell him otherwise.'

She and Catherine giggle like two naughty schoolgirls.

Sometimes they bicker like an old married couple. The usual route to church has been changed, due to roadworks. The driver has to divert through some side streets. 'Turn left here,' says Ruth, 'that'll take you up to the main road.'

'No, not this one,' says Catherine, 'it's the next.'

'No, dear, the next one's a dead end. I'm sure this is right.'

'It's not. I've been going this way for 30 years. Take the next one.'

The driver slows almost to a stop waiting for a decision. Back and forth they go, always with perfect politeness, each firmly standing her ground. Eventually Catherine wins out. The driver does as she directs – and comes to a dead end.

Annette has visited three different regions to recruit the first intake of students. She visited one midwifery school in Awassa, which offers a diploma of midwifery. They graduate 100 girls a year. Within three years only 10 per cent are in the field. The rest either go into nursing, leave the profession or come back into the cities to work.

'They're not trained enough and they're terrified,' Annette says. 'They don't want to be out in the countryside, where they're seeing every single complication that you could possibly see. That's what we're trying to counteract. Our girls are going to be exposed to that, so they need to have the skills to cope with it.'

Talking to village women, Annette learnt that they don't trust midwives because they're not well trained enough. At a health centre near Yirgalem, Annette and Solomon found a woman who had been carried by her family for eight hours. The midwife had been there in the morning and had gone home, leaving her patient lying on a bare bed in an empty room with no one looking after her. The patient had seven children at home.

Within a few minutes Annette and Solomon determined that she was carrying twins. She'd been labouring for more than 24 hours. She wasn't going to be able to deliver in that place and no one seemed ready to do anything about it. The midwife had just given up on her.

They placed the woman in their vehicle and drove her to the regional hospital at Yirgalem. Judging from the position of the twins, Annettte was certain that she'd end up needing a caesarean section. With some difficulty she rounded up a doctor to come and look at her. He agreed that she would need a caesarean so Annette booked her in and left the funds to pay for the operation. Then, believing that the woman would be safe, she and Solomon returned to Addis. She discovered later that the doctors had decided to let her continue to labour. The first twin died, and they finally took the second twin out by caesarean section. It was a gynaecologist who made the decision.

The new midwifery school will train twelve students in the first year and will take twenty per year after that. It's not like some of the government schools where they take 100. There, they do two years of nursing with a bit of O&G tacked on at the end.

Annette tells the regional health bureaucrats that the new school's program is trying to start all over again and bring a renewal to midwifery. They've rewritten a curriculum that concentrates entirely on midwifery and goes for three years instead of two. 'Sure, there are schools in Ethiopia. The reason we're doing this is we want to raise the bar and say that what is happening is not good enough, fistula is not declining. We've got to analyse how midwives are being trained, how they're being deployed, and build a model that is going to change that. And if that's not what we're committed to – something that is extraordinarily different and that is going to raise the standard of midwifery in this country – then there is no point doing this.'

The UNFPA is interested in helping with the school. They've already contributed substantially to the new hospitals. Ruth says that they've had mixed feelings about getting closely involved with UNFPA, because they tend to take over. But it's hard to say no. 'They have an enormous amount of money. We try to keep a certain amount of distance but they said, "What can we buy for you?" They bought us autoclaves and cars, the Toyota Coaster, that's the kind of money they have.'

One day after church, Ruth goes to a meeting with UNFPA officials at which they tell her they'll be willing to equip all of the midwifery centres.

You could argue that the midwifery school will make a negligible difference in a country the size of Ethiopia. You could have argued the same thing when Reg and Catherine first began repairing fistulas. And just look at how that ended up.

Mark Bennett believes the key to success will be to start in a small way, in a limited zone, so that they can see the impact of what they do. If they can demonstrate that midwives are making a difference and write papers about it, then they will generate interest from people such as UNFPA, WHO and hopefully the Ethiopian government. When he was with CMS he learnt a mantra which he thinks applies perfectly: start in a small way, make sure you invest in the right people and commit a lot to prayer.

'The community knows that childbirth is a dangerous thing,'

Mark says, 'but winning the confidence of the community and then getting the referral process to work, those are the key things. We're not going to save the women of the country overnight, but I think we can start to make a difference in small areas and then win the support of others.'

When the midwifery school opens, it will be Catherine Hamlin's crowning achievement. From their modest beginning in 1959, she and Reg – and, following Reg's death, Catherine alone – have built a world-class medical institution, with an excellent reputation for surgery and training. Prevention is the logical final step.

CHAPTER 26

An unlikely thing has been happening in recent years. Fistula has become fashionable. Celebrities, congressmen and women, important aid agencies, the UN, have suddenly become enamoured of the cause. Reg Hamlin would find it all a bit hard to believe.

In May 2004 the American trustees organised a gala fund-raiser in New York which was attended by 500 wealthy and influential people. Catherine was the guest of honour; among the luminaries who spoke was Nane Annan, wife of the then secretary-general of the UN, Kofi Annan. The gala raised more than $160,000.

An American production company has made a big-budget documentary centred around the hospital, called *A Walk to Beautiful*. It premiered in May 2007 at the San Francisco International Film Festival, and won the audience award out of a field of 200 films.

Among the celebrities to take up the cause are the Ethiopian-born supermodel Liya Kebede. A *Vogue* cover girl and the first black face for Estée Lauder, she is an ardent campaigner. The singer Natalie Imbruglia is another. In November 2006 she hosted a benefit in London which raised more than $1 million for

UNFPA's Campaign to End Fistula.

UNFPA's involvement has meant that at last there is some serious money being devoted to the problem of obstetric fistula. In the first year of the campaign 150 women in Chad received surgery. In 2005 during a 'Fistula Fortnight' in northern Nigeria, Nigerian surgeons teamed with volunteer doctors from the US and UK to operate on 500 women. One hundred local health providers were trained in fistula surgery, post-operative care and counselling. The world's fifth dedicated fistula hospital (after those in Ethiopia) is operating in Sierra Leone. All over Africa and Asia, the number of doctors who have had training in fistula surgery is increasing.

In the world of international aid, fashions tend to come and go. If – when – attention turns elsewhere, Catherine hopes that interest being earned by the future fund will be enough to cater to the ongoing needs of the hospital. The separate trusts in the US, Japan, UK, Sweden, Australia and New Zealand have come together to form Hamlin Fistula International. Mark Bennett believes that it is important for all the trusts to start planning financially together as a single international body, rather than piecemeal. Money that is in excess of current needs is channelled into the future fund.

The future fund is held in a bank account in Switzerland, as Catherine explained to me in her own unique style one day. 'It's managed by a nice man who's the son of David Barnsdall, a friend of Stuart Abrahams, who's an accountant in Sydney. His son lives in Switzerland. We often ask people if they'd like to contribute to the future, especially if they leave things in their will.

'We have to really work on the fund in Switzerland and try to get more people excited about it. We're getting the interest coming from it, so it's doing some good now. But it will do much better in the future if we can build it up to twenty or 30 million. If I could get hold of Bill Gates . . . I'm sure if he came here, or even his wife, that would help. She's very sympathetic. I saw a picture of her in India working amongst the poor. So it would be good if we could get hold of them.'

A couple of days ago Amina went home, with instructions to return in six months' time if her incontinence has not improved. The ultrasound had returned good news. Her uterus was intact. I had to be away from the hospital on the day she left. I wish I'd been there to wish her well.

Leteabazgi has left, too, also with instructions to return if she needs to. Poor Leteabazgi, so timid, so unprepared for the adversity which will surely be her lot in life. She doesn't feel as if she's been cured, although she is certainly better off than when she came. I hope she can find the courage to come back if need be.

Zemebech departed with a smile, happy to be completely cured, going home to her husband and three children.

Halema has gone too. She left with her sister a day ago and would be somewhere on the road back to Somalia now. What a story she will have to tell when she arrives home, transformed.

This morning I went to see Alganish to say goodbye, for I am leaving too. I was afraid to ask how she was, for fear of more bad news. But she was sitting up in bed looking serenely happy. After all of her setbacks she had finally been cured! She was perfectly dry and would be going home in a day or two.

With Sister Konjit translating I said to Alganish that I'd be leaving tomorrow and that I wished her well.

'Thank you for all your prayers,' she said.

'I'm going to write about you in my book.'

'Okay.'

This book business is still a puzzle to her, I'm sure. But she was happy to indulge my *ferenji* foibles. Gracious to the last.

Alganish was looking forward to seeing her kids. I fear that she's probably going to do it tough when she goes home.

I squeezed her hand and said goodbye. As I was walking away I remarked to Sister Konjit on her amazing spirit. 'Yes,' she said. 'Sometimes the ones who have an optimistic outlook do better against all the odds than ones who are always sad and pessimistic.'

These women will return to their hard lives, struggling just to exist. Whatever trials they have yet to endure I am sure that in years to come they will never forget this brief interlude when, for once, they were treated with kindness and respect, and were given a second chance at life.

In the evening I pick my way down the rocky path to Catherine's house. It's Sunday, Yeshi's day off. Ruth is already there setting up her laptop computer to show some videos. Mamitu comes in. She goes around the house closing the shutters for Catherine, their regular Sunday night routine. Mamitu chats for a few minutes then says goodnight and we sit down to a meal of omelettes.

Catherine has been speaking to her son, Richard, on the phone. Richard has spent his adult life living in London, where he and his wife, Diana, have brought up four children. They have been looking for a house to buy in Cornwall. Trouble is, says Catherine, the beastly real estate agents keep gallumping them.

'You mean gazumping,' says Ruth.

'Yes, that's it. I can never remember it.'

We have a bit of fun with 'gallumping'. As with the Rooibos tea, Catherine just can't get her tongue around it.

After dinner we put on a video called *Don't be Silent*, which the hospital had made a couple of years ago. It's a song, with words written by Biruk and sung by some of Ethiopia's leading entertainers, pleading for the rights of women. The images tell a story of a young girl forced into marriage, being injured in child-birth and coming to the hospital to be cured. She goes home and the men in her family realise how shamefully they have treated her. It's beautifully produced and very touching. The song and video have been played widely on Ethiopian TV and radio, and it's used overseas at fund-raising meetings.

After this curtain-raiser we come to the main entertainment of the evening – an episode of an ancient English TV comedy series, *Dad's Army*. Old-fashioned, corny, devoid of bad language or salacious humour, it's one of Catherine's favourites. She has a collection of them.

As I watch Catherine and Ruth chortling at the screen, I wonder about the changes taking place at the hospital, and those yet to come – including the most drastic and saddest change of all. Ruth loves this place but she doesn't plan on staying forever. During her last trip to England with Catherine, she took some time to look around for a place in Scotland, where she will one day retire. Her motives have always been clear. 'I work for God. If God was to say, Ruth, I want you to leave this place tomorrow, I'd pack my bags and I'd go. He's my boss first and foremost. I have an elderly father, a wonderful stepmother and I'm fond of Ethiopia, but I like the UK.' In the meantime, though, in the absence of a Godly command: 'I think as long as Catherine's here I'll be here.'

I make my way back up the hill to the main ward. It's 9.30. Missionary's bedtime. The outpatients department is closed. The reception area is deserted, just a nightlight burning. The curtains have been drawn across the windows that open onto the long verandah which runs along the side. I enter the ward and pass Letebirhan's bed on the left. Her wheelchair is parked beside her locker and she is fast asleep. The night sister is sitting at her station down at the far end of the ward, writing notes. All is quiet. There are no nurse aides mopping the floors, no doctors doing rounds, just rows of patients tucked up in bed for the night; rows of dark faces. Eyes closed. Peacefully asleep. Safe and secure, at least for now. Occasionally someone stirs. What do they dream of, these peasant women? A new life free from shame? Friendships? Family? An absence of pain? Normality?

I take one last look around before stealing away quietly to my own bed. Somewhere out in the countryside far away from here, a woman is suffering the agonies of labour, and on the roads leading to the capital, others are making their way, with hope in their hearts, to the hospital by the river.

EPILOGUE

Thus ended my story – or so I imagined. After leaving Ethiopia I heard some startling news. Ruth Kennedy had quit. The evolution taking place at the hospital had brought into focus differences between Ruth and Mark, each of whom had their own ideas about the way forward. During a visit to the UK with Catherine, Ruth had offered her resignation. This created a dilemma for Catherine. She was torn between her close friendship with Ruth, and her respect for a capable and loyal chief executive. As ever, she did what she judged would be best for the hospital. She accepted Ruth's resignation, thereby endorsing Mark Bennett's authority.

A few days later Ruth flew back to Addis, followed a day or two later by Catherine. Ruth had made plans to take up a new position with her friend Karin van den Bosch, at Grace Village in Tigray province. With typical efficiency, she quickly packed her furniture, organised her much-loved housekeeper, Berhanie, to accompany her, and had her dog spayed. Within three days of arriving in Addis she was ready to move.

Her farewell was attended by all the staff. Catherine made a speech. Ruth read something from the Bible and said that she was not leaving the country, simply going to another job; she would still be a friend to the hospital. Then, uncharacteristically, she wept. To add further to the emotion of the occasion, in the middle of everything news came that Sister Tsedu had lost the fight against her cancer.

Of all the ceremonies and farewells that have taken place in the Bete Mesgana, this is one that Catherine will never forget. 'I said to Ruth afterwards, "It was really a fiasco, wasn't it, Ruth?" She said yes, it was. Everyone was sobbing into their handkerchiefs, all the little girls, because she'd been so friendly with them all. It nearly killed me all this, really. I was emotional. I had a pain in my stomach for days, wondering what on earth was going to happen here.'

Ruth is now working with Karin, caring for 50 orphans at Grace Village, in northern Ethiopia. She has built a little house near a cliff edge overlooking a stunning valley of parched earth and rock. As irrepressible as ever, she has half a dozen different projects on the go. She enthused about her new life in a recent e-mail to me:

I am the official proposal writer and drafter of documents and am loving every minute of it! In between, there are nappies (diapers) to change or wash, babies to feed, kids to hug and prayer meetings to attend. I walked up to the children's houses this morning with Ribka, the one year old, on my back, sat on a big stone and was immediately smothered with many wet and loving kisses. About five of the wee ones tried to braid my short hair to no avail. After a lovely Ethiopian meal made by my Berhanie who has come with me, a tasty cup of coffee and some chocolate that I brought from UK for Karin, I decided to catch up on e-mails. Aster, one of the four year olds, came with me and decided she would sort all my jewellery, so I may never again have matching pairs of earrings, but who cares, she was happy for at least one hour. She ran in about twenty minutes ago to tell me, 'Mama Ruth the cow are out, come!' So off we went to talk with the cows. This morning we visited the stream and found frogs, also four goat legs, the rest of the goat was butchered and shared with the houses.

Ruth is also helping to train midwife tutors in the Tigray region. Another of her projects involves a village 40 kilometres away, where 60 to 100 people die each year from a rare ailment – veno-occlusive liver disease. Studies have shown that a high-protein diet will help delay the disease, so Ruth's sponsoring organisation, the OASIS Foundation, has arranged a feeding program for 400 children. With money raised from overseas donors, they are giving the children high-protein beans to supplement their normal, meagre diet. They've given them tents so that they no longer have to learn their school lessons in the open.

With a small grant from the Australian fistula trust, they've built a hostel for patients waiting to go to hospital. There is accommodation for four women. They'll house and feed them, and arrange for them to go to the outreach hospital at Mekele for their surgery.

Despite the pain surrounding Ruth's departure, she and Catherine remain good friends. They speak often on the telephone and, as I write, Catherine is planning a trip north, with Mamitu, to visit.

Bethela Amanuel has taken over Ruth's job as publicity officer.

The midwifery school is up and running, with its first intake of twelve students. Its opening was a close-run thing. The building housing the lecture rooms, library, offices and storerooms for medical equipment, was finished only days before they were due to begin lessons. Annette has been impressed by the new students. They're bright and keen, and they're loving the experience of living and studying at the idyllic setting next to Desta Mender.

There is still much to do. Whilst Annette is temporarily in charge of the school, they need to find a suitably qualified midwife, either a professor or someone with a master's degree, to be dean. Annette is not sufficiently qualified, and even if she were, being Mark Bennett's wife would rule her out.

The two girls who left Desta Mender to earn their living as seamstresses in Yirgalem returned after a month. The plan had been for them to make pillowslips, nightgowns, uniforms and suchlike for the Yirgalem hospital, and also to seek out business in the community. They found that the patient load at Yirgalem was not yet enough to support them fully, and their skills were not adequate to compete in the open market.

After living a sheltered existence at Desta Mender for so long, they did not have the confidence to cope by themselves. When they returned, they said they wanted to be nurse aides. That's understandable, because nurse aides earn good money compared with most people in the community. But there are no more jobs for nurse aides. The sewing girls are being retrained to a higher standard, and at some time in the future, with more support, they will try again.

These first two women were bound to reveal shortcomings. Mark Bennett acknowledges that perhaps they were a little premature in sending them away, but he is still full of optimism about the future of Desta Mender. 'We're making great progress. There are 50 women living there. Within the next few months twenty will move off site because they have jobs, they've been trained, and they feel confident to take their future into their own hands. Before the end of the year, Ephraim believes another ten will move off site, employed with some level of confidence about managing their own future.'

The vegetable gardens and the dairy are both making money, and the women who work there are earning a percentage of the profits. Soon it may be enough for them to leave and live independently outside, coming to work each day as with a normal job.

Organisations in Addis have been hiring out the chapel as a conference centre, which is bringing in income for the five girls trained in catering. There are plans to open a little café next to the lake, which they will run. Another step towards their independence.

Recently, one of the women who had been trained to look after the cows, and make cheese and butter and market them, came to Ephraim and asked him, 'Why do I have to stay here? If you gave me a cow couldn't I go back to my home area?'

Little things like that make Mark Bennett very excited. 'If you visited two and a half years ago and met some of the girls who worked there, and came back now, you'd find a dramatic change. When we've got women who are saying they now feel confident to take their own future into their own hands, then we've made enormous steps forward.'

Gordon Williams' new medical school, St Paul's Hospital Millennium Medical School, is functioning, with its first intake of 50 students. It's been a rocky road thus far. Three weeks before the school was due to open they had no lecture theatres, no computer library and the Minister for Health had still not approved the student intake. They had a place for the students to live but no one to feed them. If Gordon had hair he'd have been tearing it out over continuing bureaucratic frustrations.

On the positive side, he's lost weight and is in fighting trim. Anxiety can do that.

In Britain, Gordon had for some time been giving all the money he earned in private practice to the London Hammersmith Hospital, to hold in trust. He has drawn upon it to purchase almost a quarter of a million pounds' worth of equipment. He had to buy anaesthetic, ultrasound, diathermy and X-ray machines, and other essential items. It's not usually the dean's job to fund the hospital or to get equipment but, as Gordon pointed out in his practical way, 'If you don't have it, they're not operating and not X-raying so you can't teach the students.'

The main medical school in Addis refused to teach Gordon's people how to preserve bodies for dissection. So he learnt how to do it himself. He went back to his medical school in London, and they explained the use of preservative, how the tubing and pumps work and so on. He bought a big supply of embalming fluid to bring back with him. There was trouble bringing it through Customs, because it contained alcohol. At least one thing has turned out to be straightforward – in Ethiopia there's no trouble obtaining bodies to dissect.

Gordon has found a house to live in and he's furnished one of the rooms with bunks for the use of students and tutors visiting from overseas.

'It's all been great fun,' he says. 'I love this country; and there are so many people here who are sick. I want to see this through. The plan is to live here forever.'

Despite his workload he will always find the time to come to the Fistula Hospital to operate.

★

Six months after going home, Amina returned to the hospital. She had been there just three weeks before I made a return visit. I was sorry to miss her. When I heard about her coming back I assumed it was because of lingering incontinence, but her notes revealed that she had been completely cured and was in good health. She wanted advice about how to handle her next pregnancy. So she had either been reunited with her husband or had found a new one. She was advised that it was safe to have a baby, as long as she did so in a hospital.

Leteabazgi, who had also gone home with instructions to return in six months' time if her incontinence persisted, has not been back.

Lingersh, the young woman whom I used to see each morning exercising her contractured leg has gone home, walking normally and cured of her fistulas.

Simenesh has also returned home, walking unaided and able to lead a normal life.

Dr Abiy, in his final year of postgraduate studies at the time of writing, now has no doubt that he will specialise in fistula surgery when he graduates.

The new hospital at Harar has opened, and building is due to commence in 2009 on the fifth outreach hospital at Metu in the west.

Richard Hamlin, after an absence of nearly 30 years, has become involved with the hospital. He visits Ethiopia regularly to help with planning and administration.

As this book is published, Dr Catherine Hamlin is about to begin her 50th year in Ethiopia. Her golden jubilee. She has

JOHN LITTLE

no thought of retiring. The only thing that will prevent her from
working is infirmity or life's end. She is in the process of handing
over all the administration to the CEO. She will continue to
do clinical work and fund-raising. Catherine delights in visiting
Richard and her grandchildren. She plans to spend more time
with them in Cornwall; Richard might even find a big enough
place for her to have her own little flat. But Ethiopia is her home
and she'll never permanently leave here. There's a plot reserved
for her in the British War Graves Cemetery, where Reg is
buried. That is where she will finally rest.

**For information on the Fistula Hospital,
please go to www.fistulatrust.org**

Hamlin Fistula Relief and Aid Fund
PO Box 965
Wahroonga NSW 2076
fistulaltd@ozemail.com.au

Fistula Hospital Trusts

Australia

Hamlin Fistula Relief and Aid Fund
PO Box 965
Wahroonga
NSW 2076

fistulaltd@ozemail.com.au
www.fistulatrust.org

Ethiopia

Addis Ababa Fistula Hospital
PO Box 3609
Addis Ababa
Ethiopia

www.hamlinfistula.org

Bank A/C
Hamlin Fistula Welfare and Research Trust
Acct No 189
Commercial Bank of Ethiopia
Mahatma Gandhi Branch

PO Box 255
Addis Ababa
Ethiopia

Germany

Fistula e.V
Neue Heimat 7
76646 Bruchsal 4

fistula.ev@web.de

Japan

Hamlin Fistula Japan
1 23 13, Higashi-Izumi, Koame-Shi
Tokyo 201-0014

info@fistula-japan.org
www.english.fistula-japan.org

The Netherlands

Stichting Fistula Foundation
Kennemerstraatweg 45
NL 1851 HEILOO

fistula@ecomonte.nl

New Zealand

Hamlin Charitable Fistula Hospitals Trust
Box 6395, Upper Riccarton
Christchurch

hamlinht@xtra.co.nz

Sweden

Fistulasjukukhusets Insamlingsstifelse
Box 191 09
SE 104 32 Stockholm

www.fistulasjukhuset.se
chistina_and@yahoo.se

United Kingdom

Hamlin Fistula UK
4 Parade Buildings
Nimmings Road
Halesowen
West Midlands
B62 9JJ

Tel: 0121 559 3999
hccif@aol.com
www.hamlinfistulauk.com

United States of America

1171 Homestead Road, Suite 265
Santa Clara, CA 95050
USA

www.fistulafoundation.org

ACKNOWLEDGMENTS

I'd like to thank Dr Catherine Hamlin for once more allowing me into her life. Catherine endured my endless questions with grace and patience. And apart from that, just being in her company was always a delight. Catherine's son, Richard, also gave unstinting help. The book would never have been written without the tireless assistance and enthusiasm of Ruth Kennedy. Thanks are due to all the doctors, Mulu, Ambaye, Biruk, Haile, Habte, Yifru, Melaku, Andrew and Einar. I include Mamitu in that list, although I'm sure she'd demur. For the staff at Addis Ababa, the outreach hospitals and Desta Mender, no request was ever too much trouble. I would like especially to single out Annette and Mark Bennett for their practical help and their hospitality during my two stays at the hospital. In Sydney the former head of the Hamlin Fistula Relief and Aid Fund, Stuart Abrahams, helped often with his encyclopaedic knowledge of the hospital's history and his insights into the personalities of its personnel. The current head, James Grainger, gave valuable comments and advice. The manuscript was immeasurably improved by the input of my wife, Anna, and publisher, Tom Gilliatt, both of whose instincts are invariably right.